FROM THE MENTAL PATIENT TO THE PERSON

The aim of contemporary mental health policy is to enable people who have had a severe mental illness to lead relatively independent lives in the community, rather than be sequestered permanently in large mental hospitals. In recent years, plans to hasten the closure of many of these hospitals have become controversial and generated sharp debate about community care. *From the Mental Patient to the Person* contributes to this debate through an exploration of the experiences of a group of people with a history of schizophrenic illness, who are living in the community.

From the Mental Patient to the Person will be of interest to mental health professionals, users of mental health services and their relatives, students of social sciences and health care, and to a general readership.

FROM THE MENTAL PATIENT TO THE PERSON

Peter Barham
and
Robert Hayward

London and New York

First published in 1991
by Routledge
11 New Fetter Lane, London EC4P 4EE

Simultaneously published in the USA and Canada
by Routledge
29 West 35th Street, New York, NY 10001

Reprinted 1992 and 1994

A Tavistock/Routledge publication

© 1991 The Hamlet Trust

Typeset by Columns Design and Production Services Ltd,
Reading
Printed and bound in Great Britain by
Antony Rowe Ltd, Chippenham, Wiltshire

British Library Cataloguing in Publication Data
Barham, Peter
From the mental patient to the person.
1. Great Britain. Schizophrenia
I. Title II. Hayward, Robert
362.2

Library of Congress Cataloging in Publication Data
From the mental patient to the person
Peter Barham and Robert Hayward.
p.   cm.
Includes bibliographical references.
Includes indexes.
1. Schizophrenics.   2. Schizophrenics – Social conditions.
3. Schizophrenics – Mental health services.   I. Hayward, Robert.
II. Title.
[DNLM: 1. Community Mental Health Services.   2. Psychology,
Social.   3. Schizophrenia – rehabilitation. WM 203 B251f]
RC514.B3658 1991
362.2′6 – dc20
DNLM/DLC
for Library of Congress   90–9029 CIP

ISBN 0–415–04120–1

Chronic illness doesn't have to mean chronic patienthood.
(Mental health worker, Fountain House, New York)

What do you think schizophrenia means to other people?

To them it means split personality, evil and being like the Ripper or something.

They've got it all wrong in some ways, haven't they?

Yes, they have.

How do you think we could change people's views?

Well, why do you think I'm doing this for you right now? If you can get a book to them, maybe they might read it.
(Harold)

CONTENTS

CONTENTS

ACKNOWLEDGEMENTS

We are especially grateful to two groups of people who must remain anonymous – the members of the health, Social Service and voluntary agencies who assisted us, and the former mental patients who gave so freely of their time and willingly shared their experiences with us. We also wish to acknowledge the generous support of the Joseph Rowntree Memorial Trust. A number of people gave us helpful advice and support, in particular Stephen Collins, who helped to set up the project, Professor Geoffrey Pearson, and the members of the Advisory Committee to the project: Robin Guthrie, then director of the Trust, Jane Gibbons, Professor David Goldberg, Miss E.M. Goldberg and Dr David Towell. Needless to say, the responsibility for what we have written rests entirely with ourselves.

INTRODUCTION

The aim of this book is to further our understanding of the social fate of people with a history of schizophrenic illness in our society. Contemporary mental health policy urges the inclusion in social life of a category of people who for a century or more had been exiled in the Victorian asylums. In this book we shall explore the trials of a group of people with a history of schizophrenic illness living in the community largely from their own point of view and in doing so attempt to throw some light on what inclusion in social life has come to mean for them.

An earlier generation of studies explored the 'moral careers' of institutionalised mental patients but the study of the vicissitudes of former mental patients in the community is still very much unbroken ground and, most notably, we know rather little about how the people who now live amongst us themselves perceive their good fortune and think about their situations.[1] That they should still appear somewhat strange and distant to us becomes, however, less surprising when we reflect that we are rather uncertain as to how to think about them. One approach to the source of our uncertainty is to ask what the inclusion of people with mental illness in social life might mean. Are we to see it merely as the administrative substitution of one locus of care for another (or perhaps for none at all)? Or does it implicate something else besides, a reshaping of our ways of thinking about people with mental illness? It may be argued that if we are to take notions of social inclusion seriously, then it is incumbent on us to try to understand people with mental illness not simply in what we shall term the vocabulary of difference but more especially also in the vocabulary of membership, as 'one of us'. In large part the intention of this book is to make out a case for a vocabulary of membership in our dealings with people who have a history of schizophrenic illness. But it must be admitted at the outset

1

that severe obstacles stand in the way of such an enterprise and there are good historical reasons why some should view it with suspicion.

As historians of madness have shown, we have inherited from the last century a 'deep disposition to see madness as essentially Other'.[2] The transformation of Victorian asylums into gigantic custodial warehouses hastened the 'decline of dialogue between society and psychiatrist on the one hand and the disturbed on the other (increasingly "shut up" in both senses)' and irretrievably established their differences.[3] In crucial respects this custodial history is recapitulated in the traditional psychiatric account of schizophrenia as a narrative of loss in which the pre-illness person goes missing, seemingly abandoned by the force of the disorder. On this view schizophrenia 'is more than an illness that one *has*; it is something a person *is* or may *become*'.[4] The person who has suffered a schizophrenic illness is someone in which a drastic rupture has been effected in the continuity of his or her biography. Suppose we ask, 'Who and what existed *before* the illness, and who and what endure *during and after*?' Some schools of thought, we discover, 'do not accept that there is an "after" with schizophrenia, only before'.[5]

It will, perhaps, be readily evident that this line of argument poses some difficulties for our thinking about the nature and status of the person with a history of schizophrenic illness whom we encounter in the community. For if indeed the person is lost to the disorder, then the individuals who emerge from the asylum under the auspices of our contemporary policies cannot in the full sense be judged persons, may even be 'non-persons', and there is seemingly little scope available to us for thinking of them as 'one of us' in the vocabulary of membership. On this reading of how things stand, the unruly mental patients of the asylum have with the assistance of various powerful medicaments merely been replaced by more tractable mental patients in the community.

Even if we do not subscribe to these doctrines in their strong form, what does seem apparent is that our most basic cultural reflexes towards people with schizophrenia are none the less tainted by them. Bluntly stated, we are not at all clear who it is that has emerged from the asylum. It is not, then, altogether surprising that the effort to attend to the voice of the mental patient has mostly been a decidedly fringe activity, for in view of the uncertainty as to the status of that voice it has proven difficult to warrant such lines of inquiry. The term 'consumer' has recently come to assume a vogueish currency within debates about the reform of the health service but as we shall see later the idea that people with mental illness have now been accorded more choice and authority in the matters that concern their well-being is a decidedly

2

suspect one. Furthermore, terms such as consumers or users of psychiatric services, though they may be said to improve on the notion of the mental patient put 'under the doctor', are none the less still hedged around with ambiguity and we are left uncertain as to whether there lurks behind them the 'funny man' from the farm or a person with whom we could in some measure identify and become acquainted.[6]

But if the difficulties that stand in the way of our enterprise seem intractable, there is equally surely now a formidable tradition of inquiry which has taken an interest in the reciprocal actions of schizophrenia and history, and depicted people with severe mental illness as historical agents rather than victims of a disease process working out their natural fate.[7] If, as has been suggested, the incidence of certain forms of severe mental disorder like schizophrenia appears to be relatively constant across cultures, it can at the same time plausibly be argued that what it means to 'live' mental illness varies greatly within and between cultures. From this point of view, what the course and outcome of such an illness discloses is not so much a natural history as a social history.[8]

At the very least, these and related bodies of work suggest that there may be some gains to be had in attempting to tackle our inherited suspicions and to find a place for people with a history of schizophrenic illness in a vocabulary of membership. Similarly while our understanding of the contemporary ex-mental patient is still to a considerable extent shrouded in a discourse imposed from above, historians of madness such as Roy Porter have shown us what can be achieved in assaying a 'view from below'. The voice of the mad people he discusses, Porter tells us, 'is one deeply conscious of having been made to feel different. Generally they complain that "alienness" is a false identity thrust upon them, or indeed a non-identity, a sense of being rendered a non-person'.[9]

In what follows we shall go on to explore, among other things, some of the problems of identity encountered by a contemporary group of people with a history of mental illness. To anticipate a little our later discussion, we shall attempt to show that many of the trials of people with mental illness in social life are usefully understood in terms of the difficulties they encounter in their efforts to re-establish their personhood. One of our concerns will be to attempt to locate the strivings of people with severe mental illness in our society within a framework that takes personhood and citizenship as the guiding concepts and to bring into the light aspects that are obscured in a framework that focuses more narrowly on disorder. We shall provide some evidence to suggest that the 'missing person' in schizophrenia is more readily to be found than might have been supposed and that at least some of our uncertainties and suspicions are misplaced.

To attempt to bring people with mental illness under the concept of personhood, required of us will be what Bernard Williams terms an 'effort at identification' in which the person 'should not be regarded as the surface to which a certain label can be applied, but one should try to see the world (including the label) from his point of view'.[10] An exploration of this type will not tell us all that we want to know about schizophrenia but hopefully may teach us something about the difficulties we have put in the way of people with mental illness and the causes of their demoralisation, and so point us in the direction of how we might think and act more helpfully.

To undertake an effort at identification requires a shift in research style from the quantitative to the qualitative in which the profession of expertise cedes to a more collaborative way of working with the subjects of research. This book is built around a series of semi-structured interviews which we conducted with a group of twenty-four white, European ex-mental patients, twenty men and four women, selected from a larger group of forty-six whom we interviewed more briefly. All of them had a long history of schizophrenic illness, and at the time we worked with them were living mostly on their own in a town in the north of England which we shall call Northtown.[11] At the time of the study one in seven members of the population in Northtown were in receipt of supplementary benefits and it was described by a local psychiatrist as an 'unpromising place to be schizophrenically ill'. The aim of the project was to explore the personal and social consequences of a schizophrenic illness and it was conceived as an educational study in which the members of the subject group worked in partnership with ourselves in helping to put together a profile of their experiences that might benefit others. To bring out the active contributing role which the members of the group played we shall hereafter refer to them as 'participants'.

Later in the book we shall go on to make some suggestions as to the wider implications of our participants' experience but it is important at the same time to recognise the limitations of our inquiry. As has been argued recently, social policies of deinstitutionalisation have largely collapsed the structures which in an earlier period appeared to bind the 'mentally ill' together as a homogenous group, and brought about a marked diversification of experience among different social groups in their encounter with mental illness and European traditions of psychiatry.[12] Race in particular has been shown to have distinctive and controversial consequences for how mental illness, and schizophrenia in particular, is identified and dealt with.[13] However, such are the complexities of experience and interpretation in relation to chronic mental illness that to have attempted to embrace this multiracial and multicultural diversity within the limits of this study would have done insufficient justice to questions that merit concerted attention in their own right.

If, as we hinted earlier, there is a form of medical reductionism which quickly disposes of the whole struggle to get to grips with the other person, there is also an opposing form of normalising discourse in which difference comes to be glossed over or denied, as though a benign regard or the force of good intentions could prise away the stubborn reality of chronic mental illness. We have tried as best we can to avoid these oppositions and to recognise the complications that are involved. We have not set out to make our participants approximate to some standard of what could be considered normal behaviour and dress up their utterances so as to exclude the bizarre or the incoherent. But neither on the other hand have we approached them with the attitude of difference. We have tried instead to locate them within the same kinds of frameworks in which we understand ourselves and apply to our understanding of people in general. To proceed in this way is not to eliminate oddity or dissolve the enigma of madness but to help us see that whatever may appropriately be said about difference need not undercut membership and belonging.

The plan of the book is as follows. In Chapters 1 to 6 we have tried to organise the material so as to allow the themes and issues which the participants identified to emerge with the minimum of commentary from ourselves. In Chapter 1 we present a broad overview of some of the key themes; in Chapter 2 we explore participants' experience of psychiatric services in the community; in Chapter 3 we illustrate the experience of a small group of participants who found themselves isolated on the margins of social life; in Chapters 4–6 we identify a number of issues bearing on how participants learned to live with mental illness over time; and finally in Chapter 7 we set our discussion in the wider bearings of contemporary mental health policies and attempt a conceptualisation of the predicament of the ex-mental patient in social life.

1

THE PERSON IN QUESTION

INTRODUCTION

Our twenty-four participants were selected from a larger group of forty-six, thirty-nine of them men and seven women, the majority aged between 25 and 45. Thirty-two were single (five of them women), and the rest either widowed, divorced or separated. Twenty-five of the group had no educational qualifications; of those with some qualifications three had attainments of degree standard.

As can be seen from Table 1, most of the group lived either in accommodation provided by the council (one-bedroomed flats in nearly all cases), or in self-care hostels.

Twenty-four people appeared to have stable accommodation (regardless of the quality) and had been at their present address for at least two years; on the other hand seven people had had more than five moves in the last two years. None of the group was homeless though three were in the most temporary of accommodation, and one but for the fact that he had recently been hospitalised would have had no roof over his head.

Table 1 Housing

	Male	Female	Total
Own home	2	2	4
Council house/flat	13	1	14
Rented house	3		3
Rented flat/bed-sit	6	4	10
Local authority hostel	11		11
Hostel (voluntary sector)	3		3
Mental hospital	1		1
Total	39	7	46

Table 2 Duration of illness

	Male	Female	All
Mean age first hospitalised	23	22	23
Mean no. of hospitalisations	8	5	6
Average duration of illness	16	14	16

Thirty-six of the men, and four of the women, were on benefits of one form or another, thirty-one of them on Invalidity Benefit. Of the others five were in temporary employment on community programmes and similar ventures; only one person was in full-time employment.

As can be seen from Table 2, the average duration of illness (calculated from the first hospitalisation) was sixteen years. In reality it may well have been longer because several of the participants could recall being unwell for a considerable period of time before admission to hospital.

At the time we saw them, thirty-nine of the group reported that they were suffering in varying degrees from the kinds of experiences that are regarded as symptoms of psychotic illness. Thirty-one of them were receiving depot phenothiazines and in some instances other forms of medication in addition; of the remainder only five were not taking psychotropic drugs.

About a quarter had some form of daily contact with services provided either by the health or local authority or by the voluntary sector; about half had a weekly contact, much of it fleeting; and the remainder even briefer contact at monthly or three-monthly intervals. In three instances contact was almost non-existent. The average time spent receiving services, including waiting time at out-patient clinics, for example, was about thirty minutes per week.

At the present time facilities for mental health care in Northtown are still largely hospital based though the health authority is presently attempting to develop a comprehensive local psychiatric service. The mental hospital serving the area has several acute wards, two 'rehabilitation wards', and various supporting departments, including a day hospital, out of which a community support team operates. Elsewhere in the town there is a rehabilitation unit with day care facilities for people with chronic mental illness and also a small day hospital. There are a number of hostels for the mentally ill run by the social services as well as hostel places provided by voluntary agencies.

QUESTIONABLE PEOPLE?

The following is an extract from a typical field-note in our initial encounter with the larger group. Ian is 36 and had his first breakdown in his early twenties when he was training to be a teacher. In the past fifteen years he has been admitted to hospital more than twenty-five times. He is now more stable but

> Sees his biggest problem over the past 5 years as trying to find work. Has applied for many jobs recently but doesn't even get to interviews. Wants to work and feels able to. Has 'appalling' work record, many gaps difficult to explain away. Spends a lot of time in the library reading, watching TV and listening to records. Lives in a council flat, at present someone dossing on his floor (also an ex-mental patient). Says he lost all his confidence after his illness, the general public not sympathetic. Gets impression people think him violent. Doesn't normally tell people he has been diagnosed schizophrenic. Three nights prior to interview, talking to man in a pub, said he was schizophrenic, man became aggressive, threatened him. Still hears voices, 'has to put up with them'. Benefits allow him to get out for drink only rarely, yet wants to meet people socially as he feels isolated.

From this and similar vignettes we can derive an impression of the structural predicaments of our participants but the question is at once raised of how we are to read them. Our initial discussions had taken us so far but now we wanted to probe more deeply into some of the issues that had been raised, and to pursue these questions we decided to work more closely with a representative sub-group of the larger group of forty-six. To throw some light on the sorts of issues that our participants judged to be the most important we start with an extract from a discussion between Ben, Frank, Sarah and Vaughan. Sarah is in her early twenties, Ben and Vaughan in their mid-thirties, and Frank has just turned 60.

P.B.: To go back to what Sarah was saying earlier, describing herself as having a schizophrenic disability. Would you agree with that, Ben, would you describe yourself like that?

Ben: No, I do have this illness that recurs, so called schizophrenic-type, but when I get over it I don't consider myself disabled. I've always refused to take

8

	this disability pension [Invalidity Benefit] and wanted to get back and live...
P.B.:	And the reason for refusing it is?
Ben:	Because I feel it's a stigma, and also I have a belief that it's not a permanent thing. I like to think that I'll get better. But that's as much to do with my internal kind of coping with it – whether I'm just rationalising![1]
R.H.:	But is that belief supported by the kind of care you've had from, say the medical services, this belief that you can recover from it and it's only a thing that comes in phases? ... Is that supported by the doctors or do they tend to see you as someone who is ill all the time but more ill at some times than others?
Ben:	Ah, that's a good question! I don't know. Given that I have medication that is supposed to stop it from happening indicates that I'm not ill when I'm out of hospital, but whether they really think I'm a bit ill and that I just get very ill I don't know. I like to think that I'm all right and that I do get ill from time to time. But I have a disagreement about the cause of that, and the way it is treated, because I personally think it is something to do with the way we cope with the choices and dilemmas of social and human life. If you just take (this is only me and my reflections on it) the various choices you have in, say, religion – there are a whole host of dilemmas there and if you're a thinking kind of person those dilemmas can create terrible tensions in your head in trying to cope. ... What you are yourself, or what you could be.... And it's the same with politics. ... So that social argument outside is reflected in my brain. We have a mass of choice and I find it's to do with that kind of observance of outside that affects me, and that's the point I'm making. It's not just like a broken leg, it's not just internal to me, there is an external thing. I think I have some kind of weakness that makes me not able to cope with that as much as other people maybe.
Sarah:	But there was a time when you would have been able to cope with all these decisions and identify and so on. And when you have schizophrenia or whatever, it's taken away from you and you can't cope with it as

9

much. I can't explain why but that's why it becomes a problem. There was a time when you'd have probably been able to cope. You'd have said 'I want to be this or I want to be that', but you can't make those decisions any more.

P.B.: How would you describe the schizophrenic disability, as you put it?

Sarah: I can describe it in very poetic terms if you want me to!

Vaughan: You can't do that! [laughter]

Sarah: If you believe in the inner man and the outer man, if you understand something about the inner man. . . . Well, that's what breaks and that's why it makes you less confident, and more difficult and hard to form relationships and all the rest of it. That's the only way I can describe it. . . . That's the thing that happens. So that's why I just regard it as an internal disability, if you see what I mean. And that's where you get all the problems of trying to decide who you are again and stuff like that.

P.B.: Do you see yourself as having a schizophrenic disability, Vaughan? Or do you agree with what Ben said more?

Vaughan: Yes, sometimes. But just at the moment things are going right for me, no problems. I don't look on myself as being ill now. It might appear again but just at the moment I don't look on myself as being ill. In fact I'm feeling better now than I've ever done in my life. I've definitely been ill before, though . . . I've had a year to get over it now. I would have said I was disabled when I was ill, there's no way you can sort of act normal . . . you're not able to do a job, so I would say you're disabled. There's no way you can go out to work, there's no way you can cope with just normal life. Mind you, it's not physical, it's more mental.

Sarah: I don't think it is, I disagree. I'd say it's more physical than mental. To me, mental is a stigma and basically anyone who turns round to me and says I'm mad – that's wrong. It's just something that's happened which makes me act and behave in the way I am. I just feel it to be more physical than mental. Your brain still

works so you can still talk, you can still act, you're not
mad or totally mad or anything like that, but you've
still got this disability which stops you from making
relationships and things like that, so I regard it more as
a physical disability.

A little later Sarah turns to some of the other changes that have been
brought about in her:

Sarah: I find some of my values have changed since I've had
my schizophrenic illness. I don't care about money so
much, and having a car and having a house and all the
rest of what normal society does. I'm content to live
my own life as I am myself. I find my values have
really changed and I accept people a lot more than I
used to before and that's the important thing as well.

P.B.: Is that something you regret?

Sarah: To a certain extent but – how can I explain it – I
think, well I can't have it now so . . .

Ben: I don't live very well, but as long as I get food and
things I'm not going to be bothered about other things
that much. That's a feeling I have . . .

Sarah: I'm sure that you become more acceptable to society,
look you're a successful citizen or whatever, that's the
only thing it means in the end – having a nice car and
a nice house and all the rest of it. So that society can
look at you and say, 'Oh she's more normal than I
thought!' Do you know what I'm trying to say? That's
why you want all these things.

P.B.: You're saying you don't bother with that in a sense
any more, those kinds of definitions?

Sarah: I *am* still bothered about it, because I still want to be
integrated into society. Now that I've come down I
still want to be integrated into society so I am
bothered. But you just have different ideas and you
think about other people, and you think about people
in Africa who are starving and stuff like that, and it just
doesn't match.

R.H.: When you say you want to be integrated this gives me
the feeling that you don't feel you're part of society or
not part of the mainstream. Is that how you feel?

Sarah: Well, I'm not working – I haven't got a job and things

11

               like that. Now I suppose it comes down to the family – if I was working, and if I did have a job and all the rest of it, they'd be happier and therefore I'd be happier – you've still got your responsibilities towards your family.

R.H.: Does anyone else feel not quite part of society?

Ben: I have felt that at times, I have felt very separate. But I've spent a lot of time – wasted years anyway, whether it's to do with my illness or not – hating the world in the sense of unjust systems and not wanting to be part of things I felt were wrong. . . . I find it depressing and it stops me from accepting the normal kind of activities. I find that difficult to explain but for me I don't see why people can't just sit down and say 'Well, these people need this and these people need that'. Social life doesn't seem to work in a very sensible way – people are involved in their own personal games and interests and things, and so it's not often you come across people that are particularly interested in you.

Vaughan: It's hard to have a social life when you're on the dole. Making ends meet. It's surprising how a bit of money changes you . . .

Ben: It does, I tell you, I think if they gave all the patients up at the hospital a few thousand pounds, I think they'd be cured very quickly!

Frank: What would they do when the money runs out? [laughter]

Vaughan: If you've no money you can't go out, you're not doing anything, you're not mixing. You're stuck at home wondering what to do next, and that's when your thoughts take over.

Ben: I agree yes, because I think you need other people to help you.

Vaughan: To stimulate you, don't you? I think you need company and you need conversation, even if it's just about sport and so on. You definitely need to mix with someone don't you?

This discussion can perhaps help us to identify different dimensions of

the personal and social upheaval which the experience of a schizophrenic illness inflicted on our participants. Each of them can be seen to
be implicated in the wider question of how ex-mental patients are now
to make sense of the narrative of their lives and re-establish a basis both
in their understandings of themselves and in social life from which they
can move forward. Broadly we can extract from them a conception of a
field of social and cultural forces in which agents confront three sets of
problems:

1 *Exclusion* designates the structural constraints which impinge upon
  ex-mental patients in areas such as housing and employment, and
  the barriers which limit the terms of agents' participation in social
  life.
2 *Burden* refers to the cultural freight which agents are obliged to carry
  in virtue of the resonances which disclosure of their psychiatric
  histories evoke across a wide variety of contexts and the ambiguous
  meanings enforced upon them by official psychiatric frameworks.
3 *Reorientation* identifies how agents strive to reorientate themselves in
  respect of their vulnerabilities to those kinds of 'beings' and 'doings'
  which are regarded as symptoms of mental illness, to account for
  them and learn to cope with them, and assimilate them into their
  understanding of themselves.

Clearly in any one life these problems can be shown to interact upon
each other. So, for example, as was suggested by Ben's account of the
dilemmas and conflicts of human agency, the effort at reorientation may
lead the agent to theorise about his predicament in ways that conflict
with the official meanings attached to such predicaments.[1] We shall now
provide some examples which illustrate these areas of difficulty, and the
interactions between them, more fully.

Disclosure and effect

A problem common to all our participants was how to account
for themselves to others. Philip, who has had two schizophrenic
breakdowns in the past and has chosen to struggle along on his own
without recourse to medication or to psychiatric services for the past ten
years, describes the burden of his psychiatric history and the effects that
he knows from experience would result from disclosure. He has been
able to secure friendships, particularly in a local railway society of which
he is an active member, but it is evident just how precarious he feels the
terms of his acceptance to be. He has gained a foothold in ordinary

13

relationships but his personhood is constantly on probation and he feels
that he could easily find himself thrust back into isolation:

> I've built up quite a circle of friends but if I didn't hide the fact
> that I'd had mental problems, though I sometimes suspect people
> realise that I do have mental problems, but if I didn't hide the fact
> these people wouldn't have anything to do with me. . . . They
> wouldn't necessarily say 'You've been in such-and-such a hospital
> and you're very unstable' and so forth, 'and therefore we're not
> going to see you again', they wouldn't come out with anything as
> bald as that, but what would happen is that just gradually they'd
> disappear. . . . Probably they wouldn't appear and they'd make
> some excuse as to why they didn't appear and then it'd be left to
> you to get in touch with them . . . and you wouldn't want to get
> in touch with them because you know the reason basically why
> they're ignoring you, you wouldn't want to put any pressure on
> them . . . and then they'd go out of your life and you wouldn't
> have anybody, really. . . . What it really boils down to is that if I
> didn't hide the fact that I've got these illnesses, or had these
> illnesses, the people who really are very supportive, they're only
> supportive as long as you're quite normal, there's nothing
> untoward about your state of mind or health . . . because one or
> two of the people have children and so forth, I don't think they
> would want to be seen wandering about with a m . . . . Some
> people are more broad-minded than others.

There is clearly an aspect of impression-management or performance
here – of how people actually behave – but it is evident that how
people are perceived and judged partakes also from the power of
cultural categories, from the associations and images that are evoked by
the mention of 'mental illness'. Interestingly in Philip's case the burden
of his history has been eased by structural shifts in recent years:

> I don't work but by a fluke of – a lot of things happen in life
> which are sometimes helpful and sometimes not, the unemploy-
> ment situation in the last few years has helped a bit because most
> of these people have been out of work and so have I, and so I
> mean they probably thought it was unemployment, I mean the
> general situation same as it affected them . . . they were out of
> work and I was, so they didn't question it. . . . One or two people
> have got jobs but still they don't question that aspect of it. . . . As
> long as you act reasonably in their company I think you're all

right, even if they might suspect you've had a problem in the past or a slight problem in the present. It's when you start acting a bit peculiarly, and I have done at times, I've felt very stressed at times . . .

The power of the cultural categories, and the constraints they impose on people to whom they are applied, is again evoked by Simon, a man in his mid-thirties, who after a decade in which his life seemed to have ground to a halt is actively trying to re-establish himself as a person:

> If I meet somebody who isn't or hasn't been in the hospital, then you don't mention that you're psychiatric and hope to god that nobody else mentions it in your family or whatever that meets them later. Because the attitude from people, some of them, they just . . . you can tell they're embarrassed and don't know what to say or anything. . . . They think it's terrible. . . . I think unless you've had somebody in your family who's had trouble, which a lot of people must have done, but some of course haven't and they have a very strange attitude toward psychiatric . . . it's taboo, you mustn't talk about it.

Sarah has been brought to the same conclusion as Simon:

> You don't mention it, you can't mention it, to other people when you go out with them, 'I suffer from a mental illness'. You can mention 'I have had cancer', or you can mention other things, but this is something that is very difficult to talk about as a problem.

She describes how when she first came out of hospital she was 'one of those types of people that would *only* talk about schizophrenia or whatever and not talk about anything else':

> That was two years ago. But not any more. I think I've changed now and I'm not prepared to discuss it with everyone now like I used to be able to. Partly because of the reactions I've received from other people. . . . People who know me now just think I've had a nervous breakdown and they put that down to depression and things like that, that's what they think. I wouldn't *really* tell them. I don't think you should wave the flag and say 'Look!' It's not right, it's not the right thing to do.

One aspect of Sarah's struggle is to achieve equality with other people but this is put at risk if she lets it be known that she had had a mental illness. The effect of diclosure, she says, is that she is at once made to feel 'less of a person':

> It's important to me to feel equal to other people. . . . I like *pretending* to people when I go into a pub, I like doing that, I like just starting a conversation with someone and letting it flow and not saying anything. I like doing that, but if they were to get to know me really well, I'd have to tell them and then I wouldn't be on a par with them.

Ian, a man in his mid-thirties with more than twenty-five hospital admissions behind him, describes what happened when he, perhaps rather innocently, revealed his psychiatric history to a stranger in a pub:

> When I went drinking in town with two friends we were in a pub and had had a bit to drink and this fellow came over and sat down and started talking and he seemed all right at first. Then he said he had a good job and had been to college. I said I was schizophrenic and he said 'You don't want to tell people things like that, they might take you out and beat you up outside'. Anyway, I just got up and left because I didn't want any trouble.

Barry, a hairdresser by training who has suffered from mental illness periodically for twenty years, feels that people's images of the 'mental hospital', and thus of the 'otherness' of the mental patient, are still dominated by the old asylums. From his account it would appear that people react in a way that mimics the classic carceral environment itself:

> Well, I think there's going to have to be a big change with the general public because they all think it's strait-jackets and padded cells in a mental hospital and it isn't like that now. They are twenty to thirty years out of date. . . . They're scared stiff when you say you've been in a mental hospital. . . . The barriers go up, all the doors slam. Same as when you go for a job, as soon as you mention you've been in a mental hospital that's it, all the mental doors slam.

Credibility in question

A common experience for people who have had a schizophrenic illness is to feel that their credibility as persons – as people capable of taking decisions, of providing a rational perspective on their situations – is always liable to be put in question. Inevitably the sense of powerlessness that people often experience is felt most acutely when they are admitted to hospital and the patient's view of the situation is seen only to hold symptomatic value. As Steve, a divorced man in his late thirties, recounts:

> You feel terrible because there's nothing you can do. Like they section you and they listen to the wife! You see, the funny thing about my case when I went into hospital, me mother were looking after me grandmother, she's 80 odd and she were poorly and so me mother couldn't get away much, and me brother were working in London. The only person that saw the doctors and nurses and talked to them was Sandra, my ex-wife . . . and she never said a good word about me! I think the worst month of my life were that January in 81 in there, I'd taken an over-dose and so they didn't give me any tablets for a month, so I had no medication at all. . . . But you get over these things and that's it. But you do feel terrible when they make decisions and say, 'Well, he's out of his mind!'

Yet even when the person may be said to have got 'better', and no longer to merit definition as a mental patient, he may none the less still be perceived as an uncertain or questionable person who is not altogether to be trusted. Simon enlarges on the wariness which he commonly experiences in people:

> They don't know what to say because it's not like a physical illness where they can say, 'Oh you have broken your leg but it's better now', they have in their mind, 'Are you going to get poorly again?' . . . People wonder 'Is he really better, or is he still poorly? Is he OK with the children, is he going to beat them up, is he going to have a fit?' People get all sorts of funny ideas.

In the same way, the person is sometimes made to feel that he cannot provide a reliable account of his own senses. Ben describes how

> Last week I got this itching on my hand, I went to the doctor and I knew I was going to have a problem. . . . It wasn't imaginary and that's the problem with the medical service. You go in and complain about things, and first of all you have to get over that kind of obstacle and prove that you are not saying something silly.

Inevitably the family is a critical site on which people have to try to re-establish their credibility after they have come out of hospital. For

17

example Vaughan describes how when he was discharged from hospital after his first breakdown in his late twenties his wife was unsympathetic towards his illness and made him doubt whether he had any firm ground to stand upon as a person:

> The family and people around me – they thought they could just get me back at the hospital just like that, and used to threaten me with it. If we had an argument my wife used to say, 'Get back to hospital!'

Andrew had a somewhat similar experience. He has been divorced for more than fifteen years but he is still embittered by the support his wife received from doctors and social workers in her decision to leave him, and feels that because he had been suffering from mental illness he was represented as being much more disturbed and dangerous than was actually the case.

Sidney, a man in his thirties who has recently left his parents to share a house with another ex-patient, describes how his father sometimes treats his vulnerability as an excuse for not taking what he has to say seriously:

> Not lately, but at times when I've been a bit out of touch with the world, becoming ill, he'd dismiss something I'd say or do. It might be perfectly rational things that I'm saying. We used to talk about philosophy basically, but if I started getting him out of his depth he'd say I were fantasising – he'd make it sound as if it were a bad thing to do in respect of considering what reality's all about.

On Sarah's account she receives a good deal of support from her family, yet at the same time:

> My mother, she'll go on, about me being ill and I have to say 'Look it's all right now and I'm not ill any more, so just forget about it'. . . . I'm still not talking to my sister, I'm not talking to my brother, because I've been ill. I used to but I don't any more. It's really difficult.

Philip describes with pained sensitivity the outlook on life to which his experience of his family since he first became ill has brought him:

> If there's anything untoward happens in the family and it slightly implicates you and you're on the periphery of the argument and if you are not able to defend yourself – it's almost like bullying

18

really – they'll get you in and give you a roasting even though probably the argument only vaguely touches you at all, it's not really concerned with you, but you'll somehow be implicated, and in a major way, in a problem which isn't of your making. And therefore I'm always afraid of arguing from my standpoint because I'm always the loser, because everyone that I know in my family and friends they'll always side with the stronger element in society even if they're wildly wrong, because they don't want to be seen ... they know you'll never win, so they'll never come down on your side even if you're right. So I realised that, and then because I realised that – and it's possibly true that most people are really cowards when it comes down to it, down to the crunch, they'll side with the stronger party – you've always got to be very careful and you're always afraid to actually state your case just in case they withdraw whatever support they've given, that's what I'm trying to say.

So for example:

I go up to my mother's for a couple of meals a week and it can easily, if I have a bit of an argument up there, the weapon that will be used to shut me up, or to move me out of the vicinity, is the withdrawal of the offer of a couple of meals a week. And then my sisters, they'll never ever come down on my side and if they do it'll only be in private ... it won't be a very definite 'I support you' attitude. It'll be a few casual comments made during a bit of conversation, but what they're trying to say is that they can't support me because I'm never going to be supportable. Because if they do, they're also going to be on the losing side, and that's the sad thing of it.

Sometimes people on the 'losing side' permit themselves to be captured by popular humour about 'the nutter' and to provide an ironic re-inforcement of their loss of credibility. For example Steve, who differs from the other people in this study in continuing to have roots in a traditional working-class community – periods in hospital apart, he has lived in the same street for the past thirty-five years – refuses the image of the violent mental patient but for all of that still sees himself as a 'nutter':

I don't do anything violent or have to be put in, I've always gone in voluntary. It's when you get together with a load of other nutters, that's when you . . .

Is that how you see yourself in a way, as a 'nutter'?

In a way, yes. It might sound the wrong thing. By nutters – it's the wrong word to use and I should never use it being one myself.

Steve has a lively repertoire of tales about 'nutters':

I'll tell you one tale which I thought was funny. We were all watching TV one night in the hospital and this cowboy on TV started smashing the bar up, and there were a little fellah there on the ward and he were always fetching and carrying – he always had his little brush and shovel out – and the charge nurse said to him: 'Clean that glass up!', and he went and got his brush and shovel! There's loads of stuff like that happens in there, and you can't blame them for having a sense of humour.

IMAGES OF SCHIZOPHRENIA

'Thinking all sorts from different corners'

Our participants had to contend not only with the general cultural burden of 'mental patient' and mental illness but also with the specialised but no less resonant cultural burden of the diagnosis of 'schizophrenia' which many of them felt had been unhelpfully foisted on them by psychiatric professionals. Sarah describes how

You wake up every morning and you think, 'Oh, God, I'm a schizophrenic!' If the doctor hadn't told me I'd just have woken up and thought, 'Well I'm just going through some sort of illness and I'll probably get over it'. But once you get diagnosed you start thinking all sorts from different corners about the illness and it just gets worse and worse.

In similar terms Sally, a woman in her mid-thirties who, as we shall describe later, feels trapped in the identity of a mental patient, says that

this label schizophrenia is awful because I don't really think I've got it, but that's what they put on my sick note and if you tell anybody, which I don't, I don't usually, but say if they got to know that you've got schizophrenia on your sick note, well a lot of people don't understand schizophrenia and they think of people like the Ripper who had schizophrenia. In fact I heard on the radio, I heard a doctor talking about it on the radio, and this DJ said to him, he said 'If I had schizophrenia would you be able to tell just by looking at me?' and this doctor said 'Oh yes, you'd be able to tell there was something seriously wrong with you if you had schizophrenia'. People would think 'Oh well, he's a bit odd or something', and I thought well, 'What if people think that of me when they see me?', and I thought when people say things like that on the radio about schizophrenia, well it just makes people think of you in that way, doesn't it, you know?

Rachel, a former civil servant in her early forties, has come to feel that there is an implied moral judgement in her vulnerability to schizophrenic breakdown:

I've often wondered if they hold it against me.
Why hold it against you?
That there is this weakness inherent within me.

Many of our participants described how they received little or no guidance in tackling the meanings of schizophrenia, and were left to cope with the cultural burden of the diagnosis as best they could. For example Vaughan was never told what he was suffering from when he was in hospital. However

The doctor put me on the dole, on the sick, and gave me a letter. I steamed it open and it said 'schizophrenic illness'.
Was that the first indication you had of what was wrong with you?
I knew there was *something* wrong with me, something along that lines. . . . They labelled me schizophrenic anyway, so I thought having been labelled schizophrenic I didn't really understand me own mind.
Did you ask anyone while you were there about . . . ?
I asked a few, but they just said it was a nervous phenomenon.
No one told you what it was about or what it meant?
No . . . I never got no clear answers.
Have you had any clear answers since? Has anyone ever told you what it means?
Well, through going to the day centre, talking to people, we've all sort of put bits together to realise what it means. . . . But no two people are the same. From what I've found out, it covers a wide area and you fit in that area somewhere. . . . Some of the

21

symptoms are the same, sort of thing, but normally they are all different to some extent.

What do you think, the general public think schizophrenia is?

To me, they look at me as though I'm just nuts. . . . They just don't understand it. . . . It seems as though it's a disease from the dark ages.

Schizophrenia is clearly not a very negotiable term in ordinary life. For example Henry, a man in his late thirties who has been mentally ill on and off for more than fifteen years, says that

I'm afraid of telling anybody that I'm schizophrenic. People find out by accident. . . . That's why you've got to keep it a secret, because people treat you better if they don't know you're schizophrenic. I am afraid of people finding out that I'm schizophrenic.

Images of evil

'Schizophrenia' attracts a number of images and one of them – perhaps somewhat exaggerated, though we cannot be sure, in this part of the country not so many miles from the scene of some of the Yorkshire Ripper murders – is 'evil'. Harold, a former art student who has been unable to find work for over ten years, says that to the general public schizophrenia 'means split personality, evil and being like the Ripper or something'. In Henry's experience of the popular imagination, the schizophrenic dwells at the heart of darkness:

People think you have got a Jekyll and Hyde personality which it isn't like that at all. . . . If only people knew that schizophrenics are ill and they have not got a Jekyll and Hyde personality. . . . I think that people who don't know anything about schizophrenia, they look on the black side of it.

Sarah describes how the person who makes the mistake of disclosing her schizophrenic past becomes the focus of a powerful association that puts in question, or even absorbs, the individuality of the person:

Put it this way, I wouldn't go out in the middle of the street and say to people, 'Look I've had a schizophrenic illness!', because they'd look at me and immediately would *associate me with someone else*. I couldn't do that and it bugs me that I can't do that. . . . If I was to say, I've got a broken leg or broken arm, people would accept it. . . . They wouldn't ask me ten years later 'Are you feeling all right? Are you feeling all right?' [emphasis added]

Ben suggests that the euphemism of 'mental illness' is perhaps irretrievably bound in with the ineluctable 'otherness' of madness:

I think one of the things about mental illness. . . . I don't think there is any kind of politician or social group that at some time hasn't said 'They are mad!' So it's a term of abuse, it's not just an illness, it's this kind of traditional stigma about it. And I must admit I have done it myself because I think the people that believe in nuclear weapons are mad – so I use the same kind of thing.

Encounters with the law

Another sphere in which mention of schizophrenia may sometimes attract images of suspicion is the law. People with schizophrenia are no more likely to commit serious offences than any other population group but from Frank's account it would appear that for those who do offend the label of schizophrenia can prove a somewhat troublesome credential. Frank's mental illness has brought him into serious trouble with the law in the past but he has been out of prison for some years now. Getting by as an ex-mental patient is, he says, not so bad

as long as you don't get entangled with the law. The past four months I went shopping, I was very absent-minded and walked out of the shop with the article and completely forgot – it was a book actually – I got caught, taken to the police station, put in a detention room and half-an-hour later they came back having checked up and found out I had a previous conviction and also found out I was schizophrenic. They took all my clothes off me, stripped me and put me in a cell. I'd only been arrested on a book charge and then I had about half a dozen people in, wanting to know about offences, serious offences, violence and rape – you name it, they came at me! I was absolutely terrified! Anyway, they let me go eventually and I went straight to a solicitor and I have been at court four times just on this. When they got to know the circumstances – the solicitor got the doctor and a medical report from him, and on the strength of that the charges were actually

23

dropped against me, but believe me the police they can get everbody.

Frank felt that because he had 'schizophrenia' on his record he was perceived as

> capable of committing anything. The book offence – a minor misdemeanour – that was put in the background and they started bringing in all these other things. They wouldn't have done that to anybody else.

Exclusion: disclosure and employment

Not surprisingly the whole problem of images, and of what to disclose of one's psychiatric past, is felt particularly strongly in the sphere of employment. Only three of our participants were in employment – and two of these on temporary community programmes – but most people were anxious to find work and several of them had had seemingly innumerable experiences of unsuccessful job applications. It is difficult enough for people to manage the burden of their psychiatric histories for themselves, but on occasions control over their histories may be removed from them and the disclosure enforced. Henry recounts how

> There is something I regret. I went not long since from the hospital to the Job Centre and I had to tell *them* I was schizophrenic. I was sat in front of the lady. I didn't want to tell them, but the hospital made me tell them. They had got a report from the doctor saying I was schizophrenic. But people are nervy. . . . There was this lady sat in front of me as if she didn't know what to expect. They're nervy because they know you're schizophrenic, as though they feel 'What's he going to do next?' It's all out of perspective.

Needless to say, Henry failed to get the job he was looking for. Just because these matters are culturally so much 'out of perspective', as Henry nicely puts it, many people have determined that the only way to get by is to attempt to hide their past, as Ben, Frank and Vaughan describe in a group discussion:

> Ben: I try to keep it a secret when I go for interviews.
> Frank: It's the old adage . . . 'When in Rome do as the Romans do'.

24

Vaughan: I think I've become the best con-merchant going!

Frank no longer feels embarrassed or guilty about resorting to deceptive stratagems, and sees what he has to do as 'a form of self-preservation'. However, he goes on to describe what can happen if the 'truth' is subsequently brought to light:

> Like that poor lad near where I live – he got a job, he was there about six weeks, and it was discovered he hadn't filled in a form, so they gave him a form to fill in. The lad was honest and he put on the form that he was epileptic. Well, they went up in the air: 'Why did you deceive us?' But if you are doing the job what difference does it make? It's just the same with people like us. If they didn't know about you, and you just walked into a room like we have just walked in here now, they wouldn't think you were different. . . . Don't let them know you have got that [i.e. schizophrenia], it's worse than a contagious disease!

People who disclose their history of illness are often made to feel that they need to make a special effort to get over the credibility gap, to become as it were 'more normal than thou'. As Sarah describes

> With normal people you have got to put on a front – you have got to act normal and you can't relax and just be yourself. You have got to act like they expect you to act – that's what makes it a lot harder. Why should you have to act like that? . . . You have to try twice as hard to be accepted, you have to try twice as hard to do something. . . . If you go for an interview, or go for a job, you have to try twice as hard because you have to prove to them that there is nothing wrong with you.

An alternative to hiding one's past is to attempt to negotiate an understanding of it with a prospective employer. However, efforts at negotiation do not generally appear to mitigate the effects of disclosure. For example Simon describes how the person can find himself redefined as a mental patient even where he makes a considered attempt to locate and describe his past within an account of himself as a viable person – a going concern – in the present:

> I went after a job just recently at a local bakery and I saw a lady there who interviewed me. And as soon as I mentioned – I put it as nicely as I could – that I had had a nervous breakdown – I didn't mention schizophrenia or anything like that – and that I was well over my troubles – her face dropped and her attitude

completely changed. I could tell it wasn't my imagination and of course I got the letter in the post a few days later saying 'Thanks, but no thanks'. I could have got that kind of letter anyway but I think because I mentioned about my illness it went against me.

Ian is desperate to find work and he describes how in the transaction with an employer he feels trapped between the competing images, each as stigmatising as the others, of 'lazy', 'sick' and 'incapable'. Henry may find the ascription of 'illness' preferable to that of 'evil' but, as Ian has learned, 'illness' carries with it the implicit judgemental weight of 'incapable'. Ian feels he has no option but to reveal his psychiatric history to an employer because

I have got to give some excuse for the fact that I've been out of work so much. If they think I'm lazy and don't want to work, they're not going to employ me are they?

He told the other students at the evening class he attends about his history:

They said 'Why can't you get a job?' and I said 'It's sort of difficult because people don't understand about mental illness and they just write you down as being mad and not capable of working'.

Ian has suffered a long history of occupational exclusion:

I applied for a few jobs when I was in hospital, and had an interview or two, but I didn't manage to get a job. I told people I had had a nervous breakdown and they just virtually wrote me off.

Later:

I applied for ten jobs in two weeks – well I just got turned down by every one.
     Did you get a reply?
     Mostly I got a reply but it was just turning me down. Nobody would give me a chance. I've applied for all sorts of different jobs. . . . This problem over a job has been going on for years. As soon as people see I've been in a mental hospital or been out of work for such a long time, whatever qualifications I've got they won't take me on a training scheme. . . . Whatever I do, and

whatever qualifications I get, nobody is going to take me on for anything.

Exclusion: poverty

With one exception everybody who took part in this study was in receipt of welfare benefits and it was evident in every case that the social horizons available to people, and how they felt about themselves and their prospects, were markedly affected by the limited means they had at their disposal. Sally, for example, describes how she does not have a social life because she cannot afford to go out. If she did try and 'get some money together for a night out' it would mean having to cut down on other things like food and cigarettes. She receives £46.85 on Invalidity Benefit and as it is finds that she is limited in her choice of food because of her smoking habit – she spends £10 a week on cigarettes. In addition:

I've got three bills. I've got a phone and my gas and electric and I need my telephone, you see, because when you're on your own a lot, sometimes it's the only contact you've got with people.

She rarely leaves town:

I've missed not having a holiday because I haven't had a holiday for about ten years. I haven't had a holiday for ten years except when I went to the day centre we went for two days' camping in the Lake District, that was a few years ago, but that's not like a proper holiday, just two days' camping you know.

Ian is on Invalidity Benefit and receives £47 a week to cover food, electricity, rent and gas:

I try and work everything out and count every penny I spend and spend wisely. I go down to the library and study there and go to the cafeteria there rather than a coffee bar. We had pie and chips in town the other day, me and my friend John, and he bought me pie and chips and with coffee it was £3 for both of us but at the cafeteria I got a beef sandwich for 40p because it is cheap rather than going to an expensive coffee bar.

He manages to get by but

I find it a lot of struggle that's why I wish I could get a job – the lowest paid are £80 a week. I would work in a factory or anything. I'm not snobbish about what jobs I do, it would be more money than what I am getting on the sick.

The connections between poverty and the shrinking of social horizons are readily evident in Harold's description of his circumstances. In common with a number of other participants Harold maintains contact with his parents but because they are themselves badly off he doesn't like to turn to them for financial help:

Moneywise there's been the odd present or two I suppose, but I don't like them giving me owt . . .
So you have to get by on your money?
I get by on my own.
Are you on Invalidity Benefit?
Invalidity Benefit.
Is the rent taken from that?
No. I pay so much rent here, the remainder of my rent is paid in Housing Benefit and Housing Benefit Supplement. I get that as well. That goes direct to the landlord.
How much money do you have left over after you have paid the bills, for food and so on . . . other necessities?
I get by for food, just about. I don't eat expensive meals. I sometimes eat out in the cafe, the odd beer. . . . When I've finished there's very little left . . . I buy tobacco, that's all. . . . On average I don't spend more than £6 a week. . . . I can't go out at all.
What about things like, say in this weather you need a new pair of boots or something. What would you do about that?
Well, at a push – I've managed the last two years – if I could, I'd go to a cheap place and get them out of my weekly amount. I'd really scrimp and scrape that week, though.
I was just thinking – it's snowing outside – if you needed to get a thick coat for example?
I've only got an anorak, but luckily, I mean, I got that anorak about two years ago now when I was in hospital. When I was in hospital I was able to get a little bit saved because I didn't have very much going out then. . . . I couldn't manage to buy something like that now, I don't know what I'd do.

Terence, a man in his early thirties who has lived precariously for ten years since leaving home, had recently moved into a new hostel. The previous night his room had been broken into and some of his

THE PERSON IN QUESTION

possessions stolen, among them a quilt cover which he had just purchased. But what troubled him much more than the loss of his quilt was the loss of his tobacco. His recent move meant that his benefit payments had been disrupted and he had been given no idea as to when they would be resumed: with what he had left he could manage to get by, but he had nothing left over to purchase another supply of tobacco or indeed anything else that he might be thought to need.

Exclusion: burden, and loss of friends

Occupational exclusion and poverty, coupled with the burden of a psychiatric record, often have devastating effects on the person's friendship networks. People who have been through a schizophrenic illness do already generally feel vulnerable in themselves, but they are often made to feel in addition that by virtue of their circumstances they are no longer the kinds of people whom their old friends would want to be seen with, and that in any case they can no longer afford to do the kinds of things – going to the cinema, to theatres, to dances – that previously sustained the friendships. Ian, for example, now has friendships with a number of other people in the same predicament as himself, but 'all my old friends that I used to know, friends I had at school who used to visit me, I have lost contact with'. With one exception, Sarah has lost touch with all her friends from university and in the immediate term at least feels that her status as an unemployed ex-mental patient prohibits contact. She does not feel that her present life gives her anything to set against the obvious busyness of her past friends:

> Partly because they're doing sales-representing or something like that and I'm not doing anything. I'd probably get in touch with them again if I was working.

The social exclusion that comes from job loss and penury, the cultural burden of being an ex-mental patient, and the vulnerabilities of the person's own nature are thus brought to aggravate each other. Ben puts the matter very plainly:

> Certainly money can make a lot of difference to what you can do and what you can't do because you certainly can't take part in a higher social life, or any kind of social life, without a certain amount of money, and with social security you can just about manage to trundle along. . . . You know, I'd like to go to the theatre or the cinema or to concerts or something, and I could

have made friends that way if I'd had the money, because friends, I think, are important to your life – somebody to share your life with. They also keep you, if you like, in reality. It's somebody to say: 'Oh, don't be daft! That's not what it means, it means this!' Because, I mean, you can get strange ideas into your head about what things are about from just trying to think about them. And I do tend to think about things – I get something into my head and I think about it a lot.

Exclusion: housing

Along with occupational exclusion, and the penury of a life on welfare benefits, many of our participants also had to contend with a pervasive form of domiciliary exclusion. The field of forces in which people find themselves is expressed most concretely in the constraints on what they can find for a home. The situation and nature of people's homes bear very directly on what they can do and where they can go, on the relationships they can strike up, on how they are perceived and defined by others, and repercuss also on how they feel about themselves.

Generally speaking, participants fell into one of two groups: either they had little choice as to their geographical location (albeit reasonably secure), or they had little control over whom they lived with (on what was usually a less secure basis). In each case, the constraints on where people could live aggravated whatever pre-existing difficulties they may have had in the making and sustaining of relationships and, coupled with the burden of their psychiatric histories, produced what for some people was a virtual void. Not everyone was unhappy with their accommodation as such but clearly there is more to housing than material provision and what irked many of our participants was the location of their accommodation, over which they frequently had little or no choice.

As in other places, those of our participants with the most transient housing situations, and frequent moves, tended to live in cheap, rented accommodation which was to be found in the inner city. The majority of people were dependent on low incomes from welfare benefits which restricted their choice to the cheaper accommodation found in these areas. In Northtown there were two main areas of run-down, multiple-occupancy dwellings, mostly bed-sits in large old houses. One area was adjacent to the polytechnic where many students lived – an area with many cheap restaurants, take-aways and second-hand shops, and close to many of the town's amenities. The other area was to the north of the city centre where the public houses, cafés, etc., seemed to be that much 'seedier' and the 'red-light' district is located. Nearly 20 per cent of the population of Northtown lived in these inner-city wards but over 50 per cent of our participant group lived there.

Largely because it is relatively easy and inexpensive to purchase large, dilapidated buildings suitable for renovation in these run-down areas, many of the hostels, both statutory and voluntary, are located here. Four of the people we worked with were living in hostel accommodation of one form or another but quite a few more had passed through the system. One such person was Jeffrey, who in common with many other people lost his home after he became ill and on his discharge from hospital had no alternative but to move into a hostel:

> it was a right grotty place. We shared three to a room and what happened in that room was no one's business. I daren't mention it to you! . . . They had a cooker that didn't work, the place was like a pigsty. . . . The bannister rails were half falling off, anyone could have come a cropper in there. . . . Well, they could have gone to town on Social Services!

At the time he felt he had no choice but to stay there:

> I had to comply with the rules. . . . 'Right, you have to go into a hostel! . . . It was terrible. When I look back on it, if I hadn't been ill and if I'd had a bit of my own independence, I'd have cleared off. . . . If I'd had a bit of money I'd have cleared off.

Because the cooker was out of order he was unable to cook for himself but as it happened he was attending a day centre at the time where he got a cooked meal at midday and in the evening made do with a sandwich.

A second group of participants were concentrated in large estates situated to the north and south of the city where they had been provided with relatively secure accommodation by the council. These outlying council estates are relatively isolated with poor transport links to the city centre and even poorer services within. Moreover it became apparent that not only were many people located on these outlying estates, but also they very often lived on the least accessible fringes of those estates in, as we shall describe later, the hard-to-let, vandal-prone ground-floor flats. None of the people we worked with lived in the more prosperous suburbs to the west or in the newer housing to be found in the east of the city.

As Henry's predicament exemplifies, it would be misleading to assume that the housing situations of those people with secure accommodation on these estates are necessarily any more satisfactory than those of people living in temporary accommodation. Henry has a permanent home in a ground-floor flat on one such estate but the stability his enforced housing situation provides him is one of terminal exclusion and isolation. In the past he has worked as a waiter and had a number of labouring jobs but he has been unemployed for some years. He finds his living situation shameful and depressing:

> I'm living in a block of flats about five storeys high and I am in the singles flats at the bottom. I've just got one room which I sleep in and live in and I've got a separate bathroom and kitchen. It's very lonely and after I've been out I dread coming back to the place because a person needs company and it's very hard to find company these days.

The flats on either side of him are deserted:

> I think they are on social security and they use them as resident addresses for some reason or other. There is no furniture in the flats, just scraps of furniture from what I've seen of them. There is a man who comes back once a fortnight or something like that. I see the lights on in his flat. I have seen him a couple of times to say hello to and that's the only person I've seen who are my neighbours. There are people above in the other flats but I don't see them either, they don't seem to go out at the same time. It's funny, I'm ashamed of living where I am because it's such a bad area to my way of thinking. . . . I'm glad I don't see the people above really. Although I *want* to see people, I'm glad I don't because I don't like people to see me going in and out, because I'm ashamed of living where I am and that makes me feel depressed.

Henry *wants* to make contact with people but shame at his circumstances exacerbates a pre-existing sensitivity and self-consciousness:

> I have cracked up in the end in the past with being self-conscious. You get self-conscious and all of a sudden it changes to paranoia and you are over-aware of yourself and other people. I don't know, you see other people's actions in a way as hurtful to yourself. I mean they don't have to raise their voice, you can think people are getting at you.

REORIENTATION

Obviously enough reorientation embraces a spectrum of concerns, some to do with quite practical considerations in coping with the active presence or interference of a troubling form of 'doing' or 'being', others with reflections on the significance of a form of experience that may recur in the future.[2] We shall allude to these issues in our later discussion but here we may briefly illustrate a number of aspects.

'An experience which I can't forget . . .'

Even where it is clearly located in the past, the impact of a psychotic experience may have affected a change in people's sense of themselves. Thus people sometimes describe themselves as feeling inwardly marked by a strange and frequently terrifying experience which they will never be able to forget and which has left them with an abiding sense of 'difference'. As Sarah puts it:

> I had an experience which I can't forget, so I can never say I am going to be totally normal again – because the experience was so unreal and so supernatural or whatever that you can't say 'I'll be normal!'

Jeffrey describes a similar experience:

> It was unbelievable what I went through. I mean hallucinations, can you imagine it, this carpet moving like waves. . . . I was looking outside the window and I saw a golliwog pointing at the kitchen. It was a tree and the figment of it was a golliwog. I looked at it again and it was a tree. . . . It's not there all the time now, but I'll always remember it. I won't forget it.

'Go for a drink with the boss!'

For many participants it was clearly important to attempt to establish a distance from what they felt to be their 'mad selves' and in describing what they had been through they sometimes applied to themselves the same standards that others had applied to them and conveyed a lively sense of the ridiculous. For example Jeffrey describes how he used to hear voices which contradicted themselves. One voice would say, 'Don't eat this, this is muck!', followed by another voice which asserted: 'Have this, this is excellent!' The voices used to instruct him to go

33

outside and knock on people's doors and then laugh at him when he did so. 'It's a wonder I didn't get my head punched in!' At the time he was working in a foundry but lost his job because of the voices. On one occasion the voice told him that his boss was in the pub waiting to buy him a meal and a drink:

> 'Go for a drink with the boss!' I'd already got the sack! 'Go for a drink with the boss!' This was ten o'clock in the morning! There I was going into the pub and knocking on the door, and they said 'We're not open yet!' . . . They were playing havoc with me!

Eventually:

> I went round the town with just my crombie and underpants on down to the police station. They called the doctor to give me an injection and the voices were saying 'Don't take the injection, don't take the injection!'

'They saw me crazy!'

For some people the sense of 'difference' we have described sets them apart from others in more fundamental and destabilising ways, and they find themselves unable to establish a satisfactory distance from what they have been through. Difficulty and uncertainty in the inner recollection and assimilation of a period of turmoil can become interwoven with the burden of a psychiatric history – with the problem of how to account for oneself to others and negotiate re-acceptance as a person. Sally is a woman in her mid-thirties who, as we shall describe later, feels trapped in the identity of a mental patient. She is still haunted by her first experience of breakdown some years previously, the terror and strangeness of what she went through, the embarrassment she felt, and the difficulty of providing a satisfactory account to herself, let alone others, of what had happened to her:

> My family had to lock me in, it was terrible, I was out of my mind with terror and horror and they had to lock me in the house, and I thought that they were going to lock me in this room full of giant spiders and you can imagine if you believed that you'd be out of your mind with terror, wouldn't you? Well, that's what I was like really you know . . . and once I got out, I got out of the back door and ran up the street, and I remember seeing all these people at the bus stop and I was running up the street and my brother ran after me and brought me back and I remember

thinking after I'd recovered from my breakdown, I remember thinking 'Oh, all those people saw me crazy running up the street'. I felt right embarrassed about it. So that's what it was. I was just in a state of terror and fear all the time.

'Something there in me'

The vulnerability which people describe can be variously experienced as painful (as, for example, with Henry above) or as potentially creative (see Ben below), sometimes by the same people under different circumstances, but in each case may culminate in forms of experience over which the person comes to lose control and to feel put upon or assaulted. Three or four of the participants in this study suffered the degree and regularity of internal impingement which Harold, who lives in a self-care hostel, describes in the following exchange:

Can you perhaps tell me the last time you were in hospital? How long ago was that?

Last year on odd days, just overnight . . . about six times last year – no not six times, four times. Two times I was just in for the weekend, a couple of days, and the other times just the odd day. The only reason I was there was to get a rest.

What was happening with you to make you feel you needed a rest?

I don't know. . . . There is something there in me . . . some part of me, probably not really in me but something there, which is putting me, makes me get to hospital eventually. It's as if someone's putting me through an obstacle race or something and the further I go the higher the obstacles will get. . . . I'm right now convinced, I don't know what it is, but there's something which is wanting me to get to hospital.

Why hospital?

It's where I go . . .

Are you suggesting that you can't win in the end, that the obstacles are getting higher all the time?

I can't win as far as it goes at the moment. I *will* have won if I don't go into hospital at all this year.

Is that the illness you're fighting against?

It can be part of the illness, it is, I will agree. I'm not trying to compete with anyone . . .

Above all Harold has to contend with voices which 'usually question, but not always, sometimes they make statements. There's quite a lot of difference'. As to what the voices say

> depends on which voice it is. . . . It can be disturbing at times. . . .
> Sometimes it get me angry. . . . It can be disturbing at times but
> other times I can have a conversation with them, sometimes have
> a conversation going and . . . but . . . I don't really want to
> converse with it, I'd rather not hear it at all. Sometimes they
> converse with me just as strong as. . . . It can be dangerous at
> times. . . . In town, for instance, I can have the bloody thing in
> my ears when I'm crossing the road or whatever – I have to keep
> pretty cool and try and ignore it, and then when I cross the road I
> try to school it into some kind of way of peace of mind so I can
> get to the bus stop and get to the hospital. . . . There's been times
> when I have had trouble getting there.
> Are you in a kind of battle with the voices at times?
> Sometimes. It's a battle all right – it's like a war.

Nevertheless Harold normally manages to get the better of them:

> Sometimes the voices, I get talking to them . . . we have this
> conversation . . . and I'm just talking. . . . It's a struggle to get it
> right again, but it doesn't have any command over me.

'Strange but nevertheless relevant . . .'

In their efforts to clarify and negotiate their own understandings of their experience some participants found themselves in conflict with what they judged to be the official views of such experience.

Particularly was this so in their attempt to assert some value, or 'relevance' in Ben's word, in what is commonly taken for a meaningless or wasted form of experience. Sometimes where on the face of it participants adopted an official perspective, closer attention to what was said disclosed an ambiguity. So, for example, although Sarah describes herself as suffering from a 'schizophrenic disability' at the same time she recounts how she is 'guilty of enjoying' her schizophrenic experience. Her use of the term 'disability' here introduces an ambiguity as between a naturalistic account of the effect of an illness, and a culture-bound description of what a particular form of experience has come to signify in a given time and place, in this case the transformation of an aptitude for a form of pleasure into an attribution of disability.

The question of value or relevance is keenly felt in the clash that Ben

36

perceives between his own explanations and what he takes for the reductive materialism of psychiatric professionals. Ben sees his vulnerability to schizophrenia as definitively part of what he most values in himself, which he identifies as a form of sensitivity that under stress may tip over into something that he cannot control. On Ben's view of it schizophrenia is not so much an alien intrusion upon his psychological well-being as an exaggeration and distortion of valued ways of feeling and thinking, and his explanations draw him back to the integrity of a form of experience that he finds himself unable to master but that were he a creative writer or artist he would be able to represent in pictures or words. What he and other mental patients experience in their strange thoughts, he argues,

> is the actual raw material that goes into making the art, so as a person I am experiencing things that make people do creative things.

This form of experience may, he agrees, contain 'an illness factor' yet while

> it puts a maybe strange view on life, it is nevertheless something relevant. I'm just reading Dante's *Inferno* at the moment. You can't get much stranger! So that's how I feel mental patients are different in the sense that they are experiencing that very thing that you might try and represent in words and things. I've explained it, and you might attempt to draw a picture about it.

2

COMMUNITY MENTAL PATIENTS?

INTRODUCTION

For many people the experience of admission to hospital, and of being deemed a mental patient, delivers a considerable shock to their sense of their own powers and judgements. So, for example, at a certain point in his stay in hospital, Simon's psychiatrist proclaimed him to be a paranoid schizophrenic and this had, apparently, rather little effect on Simon's self-confidence:

> Well, it were pretty knocked already being in hospital! That's like you've been put in a loony bin, in rubbish bin sort of thing. . . . It's sort of the worst place to be. . . . I don't think anything could have knocked my self-confidence any more at that time. . . . I was very low at the time. . . . It *makes* you low just being in the place and *knowing* you're in the place.

From our illustrations in Chapter 1 of the field of forces in which agents have to try and find their way in social life, it is evident that though people may in an important sense feel 'better' after a period in hospital the treatment they have received will not of itself help them to pick up the pieces of their lives again and restore their confidence in themselves as viable participants in social life. The task of reconstitution that confronts them is considerable and as we have seen they may easily be relegated to the margins of social life and brought to regard themselves as some sort of social rubbish.

How then did our participants set about the task of re-establishing themselves and attempt to resist demoralisation, and what assistance did they receive in doing so? A crucial dimension of the field of forces in which agents find themselves which we have not so far considered are

38

specialised psychiatric services in the community. In this chapter we shall examine how agents assess, and negotiate, their relationships to these services. For example what sorts of conflicts arose between agents' strategic concerns and professional ideologies about how ex-mental patients should conduct themselves? As we shall go on to explore, services proved helpful in certain respects but much less so in others. Most importantly, the majority of our participants were unwilling to be incorporated in a service system in which their social identities appeared to be defined by their psychiatric histories. Because psychiatric services were generally described by participants as a system in which they had conferred on them the status of mental patient, in what follows we shall refer at points to the 'community mental patient' or CMP system.

THE STRUGGLE FOR VALUE

In order to grasp how our participants assess services we need first to understand some of their strategic concerns a little more clearly. Bob, a former polytechnic student in his early thirties, points to an important dimension when he describes what it is like to face a new day within the protective containment that his experience of service affords him:

> It's awful. I'm very bored. I go down to the MIND centre quite a bit and help in the coffee bar. I go down there to meet other people who are schizophrenic or epileptic or problems like that. I run the shop for them on a Friday, I go and see my friends, I listen to the radio a lot and read quite a lot. I go to the Job Centre. . . . I find it a very inadequate existence at the moment. I could do with a sense of purpose, of actually doing something . . . I've got nothing to get up in the morning for, it's a matter of somehow passing the day, day to day, and it's very depressing. . . . That's why more challenge, and more stress in that sense, would do me good not harm.

From accounts of boredom like this it is plain that what agents complain about is not that they do not have anything to do but that they do not have anything *useful* to do. A characteristic statement from our participants was

> I want to feel that I'm working on something that is useful to somebody.

For Bob and others, to be 'actually doing something' is to be engaged in an activity that they judge to be purposive. The crucial variable, therefore, is meaning and purpose as the agent conceives it. As Ben describes, a common experience for ex-mental patients is to find themselves negatively defined by their exclusion from any form of meaningful role:

> If you get classified as schizophrenic it becomes a kind of role in a sense – rather than being an artist, say, or somebody in society. If you are unemployed you are poor and you haven't actually got a clear identifiable role and then you do get this kind of problem. I know I wasn't really sure what I was in that sense and that seems to come as much from the social problems as anything. . . . A lot of my difficulties come from that rolelessness. When somebody asks me what I do or what are you there is no definite answer – 'I'm just unemployed', or I could say 'I'm an ex-mental patient'.

To be without a valued social role is to be made to feel useless. Sarah, for example, thinks that people see her as 'a pretty useless person':

> It's that feeling of being *useless* that bugs me more than anything. . . . I think people brand me as useless. . . . The only skill I've got is like talking to people and making them feel they're not the only one, or cheering them up, or making them feel a bit better. That's the only skill I've got, that's the only way that I can say 'Well, I'm helping someone', doing something that's a bit important.

Our participants were persistently haunted by doubts about their worth. As Philip puts it, 'You never actually conquer this problem', and regardless of what is achieved the struggle for value always has to be renewed. The 'useful' is generally defined as the socially valued but Sidney, for example, conceives it in more private terms, in the sense of self-improvement:

> I consider something like playing chess is helping me to improve my concentration. I feel as if I'm doing something useful playing chess or playing the guitar because I am improving myself in some small way.

Regardless of how it is defined, however, it is evident that agents evaluate the activities that they are engaged in, or the options that confront them, in terms of some conception of the narrative of a valued life. Simon conveys this sense of self-interrogation when he says of his experiences at a rehabilitation centre that '*You could never tell yourself* that you were doing a job, doing that . . .'.

It is against the background of this evaluative activity of self-accounting – of what people feel able to tell themselves about what they are doing – that we need to examine the perspectives of our participants on psychiatric services. We shall now provide some examples of the difficulties that people experienced in negotiating their relationships to such services and in making a stand that reflected their strategic concerns. As we shall see, agents find themselves in a field thick with dilemmas and ambiguities in which the choice of direction is rarely obvious.

'A DEAD-END SORT OF JOKE'

After they were first discharged from hospital several of our participants felt that they had no alternative but to permit themselves to be conscripted into the CMP system. For example Simon came to see the CMP system as a punishment with the threat of something worse if he failed to comply with what was required of him:

> They say 'You're going to do this if you don't do that! . . You're going to do this job if you don't do as you're told', sort of thing. They do that with the ECT in some of the hospitals. They say 'If you don't do as you're told then it's ECT for you tomorrow'. Mind you, you don't know whether they mean it but they never laugh when they say it.

After Jeffrey was discharged from hospital he was dispatched to what he was told was a sheltered work-scheme in a local factory:

> You have to abide by the rules really. . . . You see, when they say, 'Righto then, we want you to go down to the wire-works' . . . well, I had no choice, I had to go.

He didn't like what he found there:

> I reckoned I should have had the same amount of money as the workers were getting down there. . . . We only got £4 a week. So I just told my psychiatrist, 'It's just sheer exploitation, you're not going to get me down there unless they pay me a decent wage' . . . Well, I understand that they can't pay you more than £4 but I don't see why you should be exploited by the firm for only £4 a week. . . . It shouldn't be allowed.

The work involved

41

bits of wire, constructing wire to make these wash-stands – you've seen them in Marks & Spencers, stands to hang clothing on – and boxing utensils up in cardboard boxes. . . . So you're doing that, and carrying to and fro, and getting on to the conveyor belt and taking boxes off and loading them on to the van. . . . Well, if you got outside help they'd have to pay a minimum of £20 a week to start with, that's even a part-timer. . . . You need someone there when you're on a conveyor belt and you're on the lorry. You have a chain to take them off because they're coming at you all the time. It's a bit like a mail order firm if you're with me. . . . Mainly what you're doing, you're loading boxes on to carriers and then getting them on to the conveyor belt and then from the conveyor belt on to the lorries. . . . That can go on for at least four hours.

Jeffrey and six or seven other ex-patients used to work from nine through to four, with an hour off at dinner time. He stuck the job for two years because he was frightened that if he rebelled he would be refused his sick note. He has learned from experience:

Now you know the ropes it's a bit different. Because you see a psychiatrist, you go to the doctor, and they automatically give you a thirteen-week sick note.

If he had known what was involved he would, he says, never have agreed to take on the job at the wire-works for £4 a week. On the other hand

I'd go down there now for £20 a week. If they paid me £20 a week I'd work as hard as I could.

After he left the wire-works he agreed to attend a rehabilitation centre:

The jobs there are boring to be honest with you. . . . There's a workroom – that's wood, making chairs – but apart from the workroom, if you're not interested in that, well what they do they have envelopes and you put them in stacks of ten and you put them to one side and you're counting them and you do it in a rotation, and that's what you're doing. And another job is putting pins in a kind of comb, a steel comb, I don't know what they're for. . . . And then there's stair clips, putting a piece of wire through a kind of half circle of metal and twining them at the top end. . . . All boring jobs! You want to go up there, it's quite an eye-opener!

Jeffrey attended the centre for three years by which time he was

> a bit fed up with it. So I decided to leave. Then the doctor gave
> me the option of going to a Social Services day centre, but all
> they do there is drink tea and talk. That's all they do. They don't
> do anything constructive.

Jeffrey now feels that if you spend too much time in the CMP system
you can 'become like the people there yourself' and that 'you're better
off if you're outside'.

Simon also attended the same rehabilitation centre for a period. He
describes how he found himself

> taking little sticky tabs off an X-ray file over and over again all day
> long . . . it was just soul-destroying. You could never tell yourself
> you were doing a job doing that. . . . It never felt like work. . . . It
> felt like a dead-end sort of joke, almost. . . . A living joke sort of
> thing, doing that.

Andrew, a 47-year-old man who has been unemployed for ten years
and now lives in a self-care hostel, describes how he was given little or
no choice over attending the rehabilitation unit:

> They just sent me, you know, from hospital. I was there two
> months before I came here. Dr Wilkins suggested it. He said
> 'You're going to the rehab tomorrow, there'll be a taxi at 9.30'. I
> got showed round, and he said 'You start a week next Monday'.
> So I had to start.

Prior to his last admission to hospital, Andrew lived alone for about
thirteen years and by his own account had been able to cook for himself
and manage his house well enough were it not for the fact that
loneliness had got the better of him and led to a deterioration in his
situation. He still identifies loneliness as his major problem but to his
incredulity has discovered recently that the staff at the rehabilitation unit
judge that his need is to be taught how to cook:

> *They* seem to think that I need a refresher course, so they've put
> me in the kitchen.

Nevertheless he finds the kitchen preferable to his previous line of work
at the unit which involved taking tabs off X-rays and putting lollipop
sticks into bags. He earns 80p a day for a four-day week, and 10p is

deducted from his pay if he is more than five minutes late. As he has to collect his Giro on Friday mornings – he is always broke by Thursday – he always arrives ten minutes late and his pay is regularly docked.

What do you think of the wages?
It's a bit poor, isn't it?
Do you think it's worth 80p a day or do you think you're working harder than that?
We're working harder than that, making more than 80p a day [i.e. the value of the goods]. They must be making money out of it. Otherwise they wouldn't be running it would they? . . . I don't think it's fair, other people feel the same. Slave labour really, isn't it? Nobody else would work for it would they?

THE IDEOLOGY OF THE COMMUNITY MENTAL PATIENT: 'HOW ARE YOU FILLING YOUR TIME?'

In attempting to re-establish themselves in social life, participants not infrequently find themselves in conflict with the definitions and ideologies held by psychiatric professionals as to how ex-mental patients ought to think of themselves, conduct their lives and, in the jargon of psychiatric containment, 'fill their time'. For example Jeffrey has succeeded in breaking free of the psychiatric system to a considerable extent. He goes up to the hospital every fortnight for his injection and afterwards he might spend an hour or two having a cup of coffee with other ex-patients he knows before walking home, but overall

I see everybody looking as miserable as sin so I'm only too glad to get away from the place.

He receives a visit from a social worker about once every six months who gives him advice on filling in forms if he needs it and he doesn't feel that he needs more contact with official agencies. Yet despite what Jeffrey feels to be his own achievements, he continues to feel a pressure from the psychiatrist, whom he sees once every three months to redefine himself as a community mental patient and to comply with the psychiatrist's notion of how he ought to be 'filling his time'. As Jeffrey puts it, Dr Watkins tends to make him feel like a 'pawn in the psychiatric system':

Well, I no longer live in hostels, I no longer go to these units like psychiatric workplaces but every time I see the doctor which is about once every three months he suggests I go to this centre which is another workplace. . . . Well, I've said to him that I feel I'm far better off doing what I'm doing, just going for a drink. I know I don't know a lot of people in the town but just going for a drink – all right I'm a loner . . . going for a drink, having an occasional bet and filling my time either going swimming or walking. I mean the psychiatrist wants me to come under his spell.

Jeffrey resists the pressure but he clearly finds the relationship unsatisfactory: 'You're only in for five minutes with him. Well, you can't get much out of five minutes can you? And all he asks me now is the same question, "How are you filling your time?"'

For the individual to hold his own ground under these circumstances requires considerable tenacity for, as Ben remarked, people of low income and status often lack the confidence to challenge medical authority. Ian provides another example of a similar form of resilience. Ian, as we described earlier, is a man in his mid-thirties who has been hospitalised for a schizophrenic condition twenty-five times over the past fifteen years. Over the past five years he has become more settled and he has managed to stay out of hospital to a large extent, with only occasional admissions for a few weeks at a time when he has become severely depressed.

The aspect of Ian's predicament that occasions his depression is his difficulty in finding work. Ian recognises that he could not manage a full-time job in the forseeable future but he does feel that he could play a part in some socially valued sphere of activity and he refuses to conceive himself as a social 'write-off'. And it is here that Ian's sense of who he is and what he wants – his sense of his whole life-project – clashes most abruptly with the ideology proferred by his psychiatrist. According to Ian, Dr Perkins told him that

I might never work again and I'd have to be content to be on the sick and cope and manage as best I could.

Ian is unwilling to settle for such a bleak and denigrating definition of himself and his future and he continues to make plans and to attempt to hold on to a more optimistic sense of his capabilities. So, for example, he is presently studying for physics A level. Studying gives him some sense of purpose and value and he eschews the suggestion that he might prefer to attend a psychiatric day centre:

I use the physics like it was a job. I will go down to the library and work during the day and just come back to the flat at night. I

about five hours in the library yesterday working. It gives me
something to do and it might get me a job eventually if I did A
level physics.

RESISTING 'REHABILITATION' BUT MAKING USE OF IT

The individual who attempts to resist incorporation into the CMP
system may thereby distance himself from a formal patient role but in
doing so he may be made to pay a heavy price for his resistance. Ben
describes how coming out of hospital:

> It was social isolation that I was aware of, and I had to find people
> and things to do. Certainly I don't think the hospital really helped
> in that way. I certainly didn't want to go to the North Road
> Rehabilitation Centre which was one of the places they suggested.
> I did go to the day hospital for a while but I found that absolutely
> useless really.

In attempting to go it alone and to discover alternative solutions to
social isolation, however, the individual may find that all occupational
doors are closed to him and that wherever he goes he still carries with
him the burden of his psychiatric identity. This, for example, is what
happened to Simon when he tried to go it alone. Getting himself back
into work was essential to his sense of his own worth:

> It is very important. You can call it corny and old-fashioned and
> Victorian work ethic and all that, and they're trying to tell you
> that there aren't going to be jobs for everybody, well there aren't
> jobs for everybody now and it's going to get even worse in future,
> but to my way of thinking I feel guilty sort of living off the tax
> payer. . . . You've got all the different benefits, but when it all
> comes down to it, it's the taxpayer that's keeping you and to my
> way of thinking I'd feel a lot better even if it were only a part-
> time job actually doing something towards me own keep, sort of
> thing. . . . You just feel like you're a scrounger.

So:

> I went to the Job Centre and said 'Look I want a part-time job at
> the very least, can you help us?', and they said, 'Well, why aren't
> you signing on?' of course, 'Are you signing on?', and I said not,

and they said 'Well what's the problem?' and I told them and they said 'Oh we usually find people from "that place"', as they put it – the hospital – 'can't cope with a job'.

The Job Centre then 'wrote a letter to the psychiatrist and the psychiatrist said that I could do with rehabilitation'.

So Simon found himself back where he had started. He realised at this point that all occupational doors were indeed closed to him and that the only alternative to spending the whole day at home was to attempt to negotiate a more positive relationship to the CMP system. He therefore 'decided to push the psychiatrist' and eventually

I got the choice of these two centres and I thought I'd give this one a try because I'd heard that there were a commercial section there which sounded a lot better than it used to be. And it does appear to be a lot better from what I've come across today.

Simon has just started at the commercial section and is to be taught word-processing and typing five days a week. He continues to be unimpressed by the rehabilitative claims of the centre as a whole:

I don't think it is rehabilitation to be honest. They *call* it that but they don't really. . . . They do try and find jobs for people occasionally but people end up going there for years quite often and they don't get rehabilitated at all. I think it's just somewhere for people to go quite often. But they do do a little bit of rehabilitation, it is possible.

However, despite his misgivings, Simon feels he may be able to turn the time he spends there to good account. He judges that he is being taught useful skills and

I think that if they can get us a job then all well and good. I mean even if it's a sheltered workscheme or anything at all that will give us a reference for a full-time proper job. It's a stepping-stone . . . I see it as that.

The idea of the job-reference as a device to overcome the burden of his psychiatric background is important to him. This is how he assesses his situation:

I feel that I could do a job of some sort or least I could give it a try. It's another thing convincing an employer to give you a try of course but I feel that I could quite probably do a job now so really I shouldn't be just sort of sitting back and doing nothing. I should be trying in some direction. . . . I've actually tried applying for jobs but I've got the usual 'Sorry, on this occasion' letters and it's obvious that with me psychiatric background and me lack of references and me lack of work experience time-scale wise, that I can't really offer an employer what they want in the way of *recent* references. So if I can say to an employer 'Look I've done this for six months or a year and I've got this qualification', then it's possible then. But to go and say, 'Well I've got four O levels in the year zero BC and I've done very little since', well they just don't want to know, they'll take somebody else who's got the recent experience and the recent qualifications.

He recognises that his new project may ease the burden of his psychiatric history but not off-load it entirely. To any prospective employer 'you'd have to admit that you've been going to the rehabilitation centre' but Simon hopes that 'it's better than saying you're doing nothing at all'.

Another example of someone who has tried to resist incorporation into the CMP system and instead to negotiate use of it on terms that he judges beneficial is Barry, a gentleman's hairdresser by training who has been hospitalised on a number of occasions for schizophrenia. Over the past five years Barry has resisted pressure on him to affiliate himself more closely to the official spaces for ex-mental patients in the community. He lived for a time in a house owned by an elderly woman called Alice who herself had a history of mental illness and by Barry's account was often in a bad way. A community psychiatric nurse used to visit once a week and tried to encourage Barry to attend a day centre and leave Alice by herself during the day. But Barry felt that he had a responsibility for Alice and, moreover, derived some pleasure from caring for her and so he refused to go. Since then Barry's circumstances have changed. Alice has been taken to a nursing home and Barry now lives on his own in a flat rented from a housing association. He is still under pressure to attend the day centre and still he refuses. He describes his experience:

Well I went for an hour. It was full of smoke, someone playing snooker, the radio blasting, people talking. The social worker took me down and I found out it would cost 60p for my dinner which I didn't have, so that was that. They asked why did I bugger off and I said I couldn't stand the place. . . . There must have been six to eight people I knew, the rest of them I didn't know. Twelve or fifteen in the room, maybe more. They were doing keep fit when I came away. . . . That frightened me off! What a thing to do, keep fit in all this smoke!

The staff at the centre also wanted Barry to attend occupational therapy to which he said, 'No, I'm doing my own therapy cutting hair'. The occupational therapy didn't appeal to him because the only activity on offer was 'cutting paper and colouring boxes' and Barry 'just didn't see where it was going to lead'.

Over the years since he first became ill Barry has still been able to practise his trade as a hairdresser, even if only on an informal basis – for example he describes how the previous week a community psychiatric nurse came to his flat for a haircut. On the occasions that he has been admitted to hospital he has taken his tools with him and he complains that while in hospital he did a lot of haircutting for which he didn't get paid. What he would like now is paid employment cutting hair. He has considered other options but feels they are less feasible:

> I had a go at cooking when I was in hospital, when I was on self-care seven or eight years back. I was cooking meals, I cooked for about seven or eight people, three meals a day. So I thought I could work in a cafe. They said they'd try and find me something but it just fizzled out and so I thought, 'Well, I'm back to hairdressing again'.

For all the difficulties, Barry is intent on maintaining his identity as a hairdresser and like Simon refuses to be drawn into activities that seem to him not to lead anywhere and hold no meaning for him within the narrative of his life. It is in large part this sense of the integrity of his life project that gives him the motivation and the capacity to resist incorporation into a service-dominated form of life and instead to regard services as a resource or support on which to draw on his own terms.

MOVING ON FROM THE HOSTEL SYSTEM

Another dimension of the official spaces in which people who leave hospital after a schizophrenic breakdown often have to feel their way is the 'hostel system', as Jeffrey terms it. As our discussion of Simon brought out in the case of rehabilitation, here again agents find themselves in a field of forces, thick with tension and ambiguity, which restrict the options open to them. And whichever way they move they confront a new combination of losses and gains.

The sorts of people we are concerned with often lack the material resources to re-establish their personhood on their own terms. A significant aspect of the devastation of personhood that often results from a severe mental illness in our society is the loss, not only of a job, but also of a home. After they have been discharged from hospital, many people therefore find themselves vulnerable to co-option into the hostel system as the only alternative to the icy blasts of homelessness. As Ben describes: 'I was *put* into a hostel. I was homeless and so I had to go somewhere'. Jeffrey, who was also homeless, felt that he had 'to comply with the rules – "Right, you have to go into a hostel!"' – and it then took him six years to work himself out of the hostel system. Ben felt that the hostel

> would have been all right if it had acted as a community but everybody was very isolated and although we might go for a drink with somebody from time to time we didn't function as a house – it was individuals living close together but isolated.

Terence describes the privations he experienced over the two years that he lived in a Salvation Army hostel:

> You weren't allowed upstairs at certain times. Your soap would be in your room, you don't carry soap around with you. So if you wanted to wash your hands you'd have to walk upstairs and you'd get someone saying 'You're not allowed up there', this kind of thing. So you'd have to go back down again. You'd have to improvise, you've no towels so you'd have to use toilet paper to dry your hands. I managed to get soap most of the time. . . . I don't know how I did it, but I managed to sort of go to the toilet whenever I could get up to my room. It was that kind of. . . . Once I was interrupted in the toilet by the staff.

Ben, Jeffrey and Terence had, generally speaking, a bad experience of the hostel system but some people value the protection and support that the hostel affords them. This was true in Sarah's case, for example. For the first two years after leaving hospital Sarah lived in a self-care hostel where she cooked for herself but nevertheless had the support of other people in the same predicament as herself and a weekly visit from a social worker. She liked the other people she was living with but nevertheless there came a point where she felt that it was time she 'moved on', as she put it, and she has recently found a flat of her own. The formative experience for her in this respect was her contact with other people at the day centre she attends. Between them they developed a shared understanding of what it meant to 'move forward':

I wanted to be on a par with them. That's probably why I did it. Get out of hostels and getting my own flat and everything.

While in the short term Sarah valued the protection that the hostel afforded her, she also experienced it as a violation in that it seemed to her to publicise – a place that was publicly known as a hostel for the mentally ill – what she held to be a private matter:

Every time you stepped out of the door, people know what kind of place it was, that's how I felt about it.

Her new flat therefore provides her with more privacy, in the double sense of providing her with a space that is all her own and of permitting her more control over what to reveal of her private life. So, for example, when she lived in the hostel she felt awkward about inviting people she met in the pub back for coffee because of the inevitable questions that would arise. She now feels more confident:

I'm more able to invite people back without having the problems of explaining why I'm living there.

Simon also lived in a hostel for two years and his experience was rather similar to Sarah's:

It was very well decorated and furnished . . . the people there, every one of them were brilliant people. . . . I could get on very easily with them.

However:

About a year ago, just over a year ago, I left there because quite frankly the rent was too high. It was £33 a week and I was having difficulty in finding my share of it and I worked out very easily that I'd be a heck of a lot better in a bed-sitter, so I got one at £15 a week.

Simon, Sarah and Jeffrey chose to take themselves out of the hostel system but they all recognise that they were forced to pay a price for their decision. Part of that price is loneliness. Jeffrey, for example, now lives in a housing association flat on the top floor of a converted Victorian house and while he has a small number of social contacts elsewhere in the town the only contact he has in the house is with the old lady who lives next door to him for whom he carries the milk upstairs. Sarah, while she is pleased to have made the move, still has

51

apprehensions about it. From within her protected situation in the hostel she found it difficult to envisage what it would be like living on her own:

> I have days when I like it and days when I don't. . . . It'll be interesting to see what happens. I'm not one hundred per cent happy with this place but what other choices have I got?

Simon doesn't know anybody where he lives now:

> Everybody seems to keep themselves to themselves. I've only ever spoken to one person and he seemed very sort of abrupt and didn't seem to want to really know. It isn't the same as the hostel where you shared communal facilities like the TV room, the laundry room and the kitchen – the main kitchen – so you tend to mix a bit: there is one or two prefer to keep themselves to themselves but usually people tend to mix pretty well. And it's completely different when you move out of a place like that, everybody just sort of shuts the door and that's it, bars are up and you never see them. It's a shame really.

For Simon, as for Jeffrey and Sarah, the transition out of the hostel system is in many ways a painful experience in which people have to contend with significant loss of contact and support. Yet nevertheless they all feel that they have 'moved on', and that they are now much more able to live their lives on their own terms. If he had to choose again between a hostel and an independent flat, Simon would still opt for independence. He puts plainly what is, very largely, a shared view:

> I would choose to stay where I am because I didn't like the idea of being connected with the hospital. I know it sounds daft but I've always regarded the hospital as being like Colditz, . . . the sort of place that you don't want to be, and I also have the general idea that I want to eventually break off from the whole system and be totally independent. In every other sense than that, the hostel situation were a good one, it's just the thing at the back of your mind where you sort of say 'This is part of the hospital, I'm still really in the system, and therefore I'm not really anywhere near being better' sort of thing.

To feel part of the system, in this sense, is to feel less than a person:

> It's a bit demoralising. . . . You're sort of tied to the strings of the hospital, the apron strings of the hospital I suppose you could say,

you're being treated like a child really, and you prefer to think 'Well, I'd like to be independent and this is OK temporarily but I want to move on eventually and break away from all this'.

GOING IT ALONE

Facing life alone often places a severe strain on the person's resilience and inner resources and, at points, he may come to find that his sense of pride is at odds with his actual felt needs. This is perhaps particularly so, as we shall see, in the case of men. Not infrequently, the person finds himself in a field of forces in which he is made to feel demoralised about his own prospects, about what he can realistically hope for, and his demoralisation may then impact upon his ability to care for himself, which in its turn, may demoralise him still further. For the person to ask for help in this situation – even to admit to himself that he is in need of help – may seem to confirm the feelings of incompetence and humiliation that have already been borne upon him.

Simon, as we have seen, was glad to break the strings of the CMP system but in his new situation he was grateful for the support of a social worker in his dealings with an unscrupulous landlord. After Simon left the hostel, the social worker

> said he'll continue being my social worker if I need any help, and he *has* helped us out. I had a problem with the electricity – they tried to charge me for what the previous tenant had used – and he took the reading of the meter and said that if need be he'd get that sorted out. It seems as though I'm going to be able to sort it out myself but he did come down and look into it. And he also asked me if I needed any help with furniture and that, but I'd sorted that out with the Catholic Housing. And he inquired as to whether I could get a Social Security grant, but I couldn't. . . . That's about it really. But if the help's needed I think they're usually there. . . . Sometimes they're too busy to deal with you straightaway but they do get round to it.

For Ben, going it alone has

> led me to something which I don't consider is my mental illness but which is part of my life and that's depression. . . . I wasn't depressive particularly before. . . . So it leads to a certain kind of depression and I can lead not a very good life on my own in the flat – you know, I won't wash up and clean up and things and I can get in a mess at times. But I don't consider that as mental

illness – it might be something to do with my mental health and routines and things, but when you're unemployed you've got no external discipline to make you do anything. Nobody comes across the door and certainly nobody from the hospital has ever been across my door since I came out of hospital.

Ben has befriended a number of other people in the same predicament as himself in his neighbourhood and he offers his own observations:

I can see how they've coped the people I know. . . . My biggest impression is that they don't do very much. Why that is, is that they're mainly used to being employed – they're working kind of people – and now they're isolated and don't have anything to do. So I see them as being lonely. I know that two particular people I go and visit and go for a drink with, I'm maybe their only visitor or friend that would go and just pop in and say 'Hello there, are you all right, how's things with you?' One man, he just sits in front of the television and must have four pints of beer a night, and he's happy in a way. He's quite a good mechanic and he helps me repair my car – we repaired my car together. The other man I organised to do a garden with, an allotment – neither of us really liked gardening so it didn't really get off the ground, it was just full of weeds! – but we did do that. And I also got him involved in the MIND group, but he's interested really in playing bridge or just going for a drink. He's very isolated – I go round his house and sometimes he gets in quite a mess, he doesn't clean up and things like that.

In Ben's experience

There are quite a few ex-patients like that and that's why I think that community nurses should be around, really, because you do feel better – certainly I feel better – when you clear up. . . . But when you're living on your own – I don't think it's unique to mentally ill patients – nobody's coming round : . . it's a bit of laziness really!

As Ben rightly remarks, the problems he describes are neither peculiar to ex-mental patients nor are they necessarily a product of mental illness itself. They are, instead, the kinds of problems faced by single men in general and isolated single men in particular. 'Women', as Ben comments, 'seem to cope with it better – keeping flats nice and tidy – maybe it's the way we were brought up as men'. Yet if nurses were to appear uninvited at the doors of the men he has described, would they not feel humiliated?

> That's only because we've got this stigma about being helped –
> nurses coming in and doing it for you when you should be able to
> do it yourself. But I know from my own self that I need people to
> come and give me a bit of a push, and if you're not married and
> you're not working there is nobody to kind of force you to do
> anything and I think sometimes we just need a bit of force
> because self-discipline is one of the hardest things to achieve, so
> you can get problems just from that lonely kind of existence.

Ben outlines a general position about the merits of professional intervention in this sphere, but when the question is brought back to his own individual case he becomes more equivocal. Nobody from the hospital has crossed Ben's door since he was discharged, but would he actually *want* someone to? In the answer that he gives, we can sense the tension between his dignity and his actual felt needs:

> Ah! . . . I think perhaps they *should* have done . . . but whether I
> *want* them or not . . . I'm not sure . . . I don't seem to have an
> opinion on that. I don't particularly not want them to, but I just
> feel they perhaps should have visited me, just seeing that I was
> coping all right really.

RELATIONSHIPS BETWEEN EX-MENTAL PATIENTS

In having recourse to the official spaces for ex-mental patients, the individual is, of course, brought into contact not only with psychiatric professionals but also with other ex-patients. These relationships bring out another aspect of the ambiguity and tension in the individual's dealings with the psychiatric system. Viewed and experienced in one way, such relationships may offer solidarity in a common predicament; viewed and experienced in another, they may serve to put in question the agent's membership of a wider community. People who associate with other ex-mental patients may risk incorporation into a mental patient sub-culture and into marginalised self-definitions; the price of the integrity of going it alone, on the other hand, may be the loss of real relations of value and the risk of painful social isolation.

Ben, for example, has learned to seek out relationships with ex-mental patients who share his concerns and to distance himself from those that embrace – albeit ironically – images of mental patienthood.

He explains why he tends to avoid what he calls the 'patient sub-culture':

> It's a funny sub-culture. .... There's a certain amount of mockery in it as if they say, 'Come on, take your tablets!' kind of thing.... There's a strange sort of sub-culture there where they say, 'You haven't got a job have you? How did you get a job? You're a *mental patient!*' – because I'm known as a mental patient not as a technician or a college student or something. .... There is that kind of prejudice there and I do it myself. If someone's talking about making a record I say, 'You're not really going to make a record!', whereas I wouldn't really say that if I hadn't known he'd been a mental patient.

Ben says of himself that

> I don't particularly want to dwell on my illness in a sense – although I would like to help other people, and it does help talking – I don't particularly want to. I want to go on and do other things regardless of that.

When he came out of hospital, there was a strong part of him that didn't want to get involved in meetings of ex-patients:

> I wanted to leave that behind and get on with other things – acting as an equal in society and not harping on about my own particular problems.

However, a friend persuaded him to attend a meeting of the local MIND group. Ben has now become a regular member of the group, and here – in contast to the sub-culture he described above – he has found other people who do not wish to 'dwell on the illness' and who want to find ways of 'doing things regardless'.

> I did go along to this MIND meeting and I did find benefit in talking to other people because I did feel a bit alone myself – having experienced things and feeling that I was misunderstood. I feel that talking to other people has helped and that doesn't happen in the hospital – they don't seem to have groups that talk, everything is so individual.

Partly because of his past experience of the 'patient sub-culture', Ben was surprised to find how much he came to value the group:

> What I have had over the years is a desperation that I couldn't do

anything, but with the involvement in the MIND group and things like that, I feel like fighting now a lot more than what I have ever done before. I feel encouraged. I feel more courageous. I feel a bit more optimistic. Maybe I can get something!

Some people manage the tension we have described by learning how to move in and out of 'mental patient' space on their own terms, without feeling contained or defined by it. One such person is Barry. As we described earlier, Barry refuses to attend the day centre but he continues to value the social contacts he made at the hospital and is a member of a support group for ex-patients.

If I go anywhere else like a pub I don't know what is going on. If I go to the hospital I can relate to people. They tell me what they're going through and I tell them what I'm going through. . . . Sometimes it works sometimes it doesn't. That's how you meet people.

Bob acknowledges that it is sometimes helpful to have friends who are ex-patients 'because they do know what it's like when you're feeling off or whatever'; however,

one difficulty if you have friends like that is that they tend to talk about medication and their symptoms all the time like old women gossiping. It depresses you at times like that, you just don't want to talk about things like that, you want to talk about normal things everybody else talks about – sex, drugs, rock and roll or something, or horse racing. . . . You want to break out of that mould of being part of a schizophrenic fellowship or whatever. It does get you down at times.

In a group discussion Vaughan warns of the dangers of associating too strongly with other ex-mental patients:

It's dangerous I think. It's all right when you come out of hospital – you need that sort of security. But when you've been out for about a year you should start building your own life and looking for new horizons and mixing with other people who've never had it, even if you have to put a bold front on – a false image if you like – but you've definitely got to try.

Sarah then puts a different view:

I disagree! You see I don't see the people I mix with – I mean I'm involved in a lot of groups – as being any *different*. I'm learning from them how to cope with the illness itself, I'm learning from their experiences, and I think talking to them is really rewarding and I don't see them as being any different or totally abnormal. I stick with my own kind, and there's this feeling that 'Oh, you've got to get back and go out with "normal" people' and stuff like that – it's all a load of baloney!

Assertive though he is, Vaughan at the same time recognises that there are other parts of his experience which can be worked out only in collaboration with other people who have been through a similar experience:

Being on your own, I don't think it does your illness any good. . . . When we got together we found out more off each other than ever the doctors told us. We just pieced it together from there . . . at least we could understand it more.

One person who has a wide network of social relationships outside the psychiatric system is Rachel, a single woman in her early forties. She describes how

I don't particularly want to make social contacts with people who I *know* have had illnesses. No doubt there are many people in the community who have had illnesses before, but I would rather be accepted as being normal and mix with normal people as far as possible.

After her first breakdown her consultant suggested that her isolated life-style had been a contributory factor in her illness and encouraged her to expand her social life. She is now active in a wide variety of groups:

There's the environmental group that I've been involved in. There was a time when I was involved in a music society which met on a Saturday for singing, but I seem to have given that a miss for the last few years. But I'm still very involved in the Church and we sometimes have Saturday events which I like to get involved in and since the last eighteen months I belong to a singles group which meets on alternate Thursday nights and some Saturday nights. The Thursday night meetings coincide with the Bible study group I belong to, and the Saturday meetings are only occasional, so I tend to make the Saturdays rather than the Thursdays.

None the less, despite all this evident busyness, at a deeper level she feels that something is missing. She describes how she was disappointed to find that

> it was mostly older people that belonged to these societies. I seem to belong to a missing age group. Probably because people of my age group have got young families and tend to be married to a large extent.

So, for example, it would appear that the environmental group does not provide a favourable terrain for the development of personal relationships:

> I don't find it that sort of a friendly group, no. It's very much a formal group where the topic of conversation is the plants or the birds. We're very much a group that tends to talk in terms of Mr and Mrs – particularly at the meetings it's always referred to as Mr so-and-so, Mrs so-and-so, not Christian names at all because I actually gave a Christian name once, and they gave a surname as well, and I got this retort back about we're formal at this place, which I sort of think . . . well, the alternative is to give it up and not go out on these rambles any more, or to stick it out, and I've decided to stick it out.

Much as many of the people we are concerned with may want to make relationships outside the psychiatric system, doing so is not easy, not least because of the heavy burden of self-accounting that is involved. People may then find themselves thrown back to relationships within the system as the only alternative to isolation. Sidney describes one aspect of his experience:

> I do lack confidence in mixing with groups of people. Not so long ago since, I went to college to study a foundation course in music and I found that I couldn't cope with just mixing with people in the class. . . . The work I could cope with but I couldn't cope with mixing with groups of people. I tend to feel isolated and I couldn't compete with them on equal terms. They were branching off into sub-groups and I didn't feel that I belonged to any one of them. . . . I wasn't able to mix properly. That's always been a problem with me.

At the day hospital he attends once a week by contrast:

> There it's different, we all have the same problems, there's very

little cynicism there, I mean everybody's in the same boat, it's a lot easier to mix socially there. The biggest difference is competition. In a group of students there's competition for supremacy. . . . Some people are going to be better at doing the work – playing their instruments or whatever – some people are going to be better at making conversation, some are more aggressive than others. . . . There's a tremendous amount of competition there all the time. There's no competition at the day centre between people, nobody's trying to prove anything there.

Sidney now has a girl-friend whom he met in a night-club but with whom he had been acquainted previously when she was a patient in the same hospital as him. He would prefer to strike up a relationship with a woman who had no connection with the psychiatric system but his experience has brought him to the reluctant conclusion that this avenue is not open to him. In his description of what might happen in such an encounter we can readily appreciate the painful constraints that the burden of accounting for a psychiatric history imposes:

I might have got talking to her but I would have had to cut off at a certain point because I knew that once she found out about the background she'd lose interest. . . . It would have been more difficult to carry on with the relationship. . . . I have actually avoided getting into relationships because of the difficulty I would have in explaining what I'd been through, and what it all means, to someone. . . . If I met someone in a pub or a club or whatever, and I liked her, if I felt that she'd never known anything about mental illness, never experienced anything to do with it, I'd avoid talking to her . . . because it would seem pointless to me. I'd just stop it dead.

One effect of his psychiatric history, he goes on to say, has been to 'stop a few relationships before they'd started'.

MEDICATION? 'YES, BUT IT'S NOT THE *ONLY THING*'

The pressure to accept a definition of oneself as a community mental patient emerges most forcibly in relation to medication. It is here that awkward questions about the capacities of people with a history of mental illness to exert control over their own lives, and to make rational judgements about matters that concern their own well-being, are brought into sharp relief. One cast on the benefits of medication is given by Steve:

> By the time it gets to the end of the month I'm really ready for that injection. I don't know what the drug does – Largactil really is a strait-jacket – but I don't know what this drug – Clopixol – does. . . . What it's like is you get your injection and it's just like having a bottle of whisky – not that I've ever had a bottle of whisky! – but you feel calm. You know it's a funny thing you feel knocked out really. The stuff you were worried about before your injection just flows over you.

Were he to give up the injections, Steve says:

> I'd probably get into trouble. I'd probably get a bit excited and trouble would develop. I like to be kept tranquillised after all this time. . . . I'm not violent, I've never been violent in all my record, but I act on impulse and I think I'm better on injections.

The majority of our participants, however, were much less enamoured of the virtues of being 'knocked out' or 'kept tranquillised' than Steve. Most of them did not object – in the short term at least – to taking medication, and indeed many of them found it beneficial, but they were intent upon ensuring that medication did not interfere with what they held to be the main priorities in their lives. And it was here that conflicts with the medical profession arose. What participants looked for from psychiatrists was an approach that took account of their needs and concerns as persons, an approach in which – to put the matter in more formal terms – the prescription of antipsychotic drugs was an adjunct to a psychosocial understanding of their predicaments rather than a substitute for such understanding. Our participants perceived medication not as a good in itself but as contributing to some wider strategy that enabled them to live their lives as relatively ordinary people within the limits of their vulnerabilities, and they were troubled – and not infrequently angered – by professional attitudes that appeared to demean them and to take no account of their strategic concerns. In our discussions drugs were often invoked as a figure or symbol of such professional attitudes. For example as we shall see presently, Ben continues to take medication and feels that it benefits him but he said about his relationship with his psychiatrists:

> They just pump me full of drugs and I go away. There is no in-depth conversation.

A number of participants felt that doctors took inadequate account of the tendency of psychotropic drugs, particularly in high dosages, to reduce the efficiency and stamina of the person in performing day-to-day tasks. The demonstrably impaired capacities of such a person may then serve as a constant reminder to him and others of his status as a community mental patient. For example Vaughan sees himself as vulnerable and in need of medication and he has learned from experience that if he stops his medication he generally goes 'high and then all of a sudden I start going paranoid, to hear voices, and to feel that people are watching me when I go out'. None the less he is unwilling to accept a construction of himself as a social 'write-off', a career mental patient, and after discharge from hospital he has always been eager to get back to work. In a group discussion he describes his experiences with psychiatrists in attempting to negotiate his concerns:

> That's the big battle, the battle with the doctors, when you're feeling better and you feel it's time to cut down your tablets. The doctor I saw said 'You're going to need injections for the rest of your life'. I said I was going to look for a job and he said 'I wouldn't bother looking for a job, just get an hour or two's rest every day'. I said 'That's no good, I want to get out and get a job'. He said, 'Oh no, I should take it easy'.

Vaughan, however, was not to be deterred and he succeeded in finding himself a job. Once he started work he quickly discovered that the high level of medication he had been prescribed limited his capacity:

> I couldn't do nowt . . . I'd just lean on the shovel, I'd be tired you know.

Refusing to be beaten Vaughan returned to the doctor but the doctor said

> 'Either you keep on these injections or you lose your job'. I said 'I'm going to lose my job anyway!'

Frank commented that work and medication were not compatible: 'one works against the other'. Vaughan, however, although sympathetic to this conclusion, was reluctant to make it for himself and to abandon medication entirely, preferring to hold out for a compromise that suited his particular needs and purposes. After struggling along on his present dosage for a while longer, he again returned to the doctor and said

> 'I can't do with it anymore!' So then the doctor cut the injections

down in half and he gave me some more tablets and after about a month these tablets began to work and I was all right then. . . . But if I'd been in a five day a week job I'd have been sacked. There is no way I could have kept it. When you've got a job, you need all your wits about you . . . you've got to mix on equal terms, take them at their own game, . . . getting pumped with all these tablets you go round like a zombie or something.

The shock of the first breakdown often brings about a collapse of confidence in which patients take on trust what medical authorities declare to be best for them. Simon describes how over the years he has learned to hold firm on his own judgements.

Well at first you just trusted the doctors. I did, and I think everybody else does. In fact some people carry on all their lives doing so – you know, 'They're right and know more than what you do'. At first I just accepted everything but I think when I had that bad side-effect I realised all was not well. Then they put me on something else that didn't have the same side-effects so I thought maybe I was just unlucky and then I started getting Modecate shuffle where I could hardly move my legs and just couldn't get out of the chair. They thought I was playing silly buggers but I wasn't. Now I am adamant that I stay on this 25mg and there is no way they are going to increase it or alter it in any way. I tell them what I want. I don't let them tell me. But at first I accepted what they said and took the injections or medicine, whatever they said.

He now takes a small dose of Haldol once every four weeks:

I prefer not to bother but it doesn't have any side-effects. . . . There seems no problem taking it but it keeps the doctor happy and keeps me in benefit because if I gave up and refused medication, in theory they could stop my benefit because I had refused treatment. The way I understand the benefit system. . . . I'm not say it would come to that if I did refuse it, but it could do, and it would seem like why upset the applecart. I'm getting no side-effects, so let it be.

Dr Wilkins told him he might need to take medication for the rest of his life and compared the long-term treatment for schizophrenia with that for diabetes. However, Simon was unimpressed by this effort at the medical normalisation of his fate:

I've heard of diabetics who are able to stop using insulin so to my way of thinking, even using the comparison the doctor used, it ought to be possible for me one day to say 'I don't need this thing'.

Simon is critical of medical regimes in which medication is by and large the exclusive form of treatment at the expense of counselling and therapy:

If we have hospitals in the future, I think they have got to be changed in that sense – I think the whole emphasis has to be altered towards telling people about their problems rather than just turning them into vegetables and leaving them to sort their own problems out . . . I think generally that hospitals are understaffed and if they drug everybody they are easier to control. Give everybody their Mogadon, then they are going to sleep through the night. So whether you need Mogadon or not, you are given it. You may turn round and say, 'I don't need that!', and you are told, well yes you do.

In his own experience of medication:

I have never found it made me think, 'Well, am I thinking right? Am I getting ideas right?' . . . On a lot of medication I just stop thinking completely, it's just like being in a dream. To my way of thinking, you're not going to alter your ideas or do anything – you're just going to get medication and be back to square one. That's why so many people end up going in and out of hospital like yo-yos, because it's just medication they come for. They have medication and are mentally asleep again. It doesn't cure them in any way, make them able to work again.

Sidney is an example of someone who has been through a long period of debate and experiment over medication and has now come to the qualified judgement that it is useful to him and that he needs to continue with it. He feels that there is something about him that makes him vulnerable. He is presently on Sulpiride and he says that if he stopped taking it he would start

cracking up . . . I'd start getting ideas about such things as magic, good and evil and things like that out of proportion. I'd just misinterpret ordinary events so there would be a special meaning that wasn't really there, and eventually, well, the last time I just passed out.

Before that he was on a different drug which he persuaded the consultant to change:

> I feel quite happy with my medication at the moment. Last time I became ill because I stopped taking the tablets. I stopped taking them because I couldn't tolerate the side-effects. I gradually cut down and gradually felt better and better till I got over-confident, and stopped taking them. I thought I'd probably be all right without them. . . . I wasn't. This time I've no intention whatsoever of stopping taking the tablets unless possibly things change and I start having side-effects which I don't have at the moment.

The main side-effect of which he complained was loss of sexual interest and prowess which generated a good deal of anguish in his relationship with his girl-friend. He also suffered from a tremor. The tremor has now gone and he is sexually more active. Sidney has come to a provisional decision that the benefits of medication outweigh the costs. It is, we should note, very much a decision that he has taken himself on the basis of his own experience. He has chosen to continue with the medication but only so far as it does not interfere with what *he* judges to be his priorities.

Cyril is an ex-weaver in his mid-fifties who, since his wife died some years ago, now cares single-handedly for his severely handicapped sister-in-law. Looking after Sylvia demands his constant attention but he has recently been put on a new drug with, it would seem, little or no effort to monitor its effects. He describes how he now feels 'doped' most of the time:

> Do you put that down to the drug?
> Oh yes.
> But are you happy to go on taking it for the time being?
> So long as the doctor think's it necessary – I'm in his hands. I can't say, 'Now I'm going to stop all medication', because I haven't a clue about what's going on.
> What do you think would happen if you stopped medication – at a guess?
> I'd have a breakdown – I think I would have a breakdown because my body has got used to all this medication.

Despite his faith in medical expertise Cyril is unhappy about his relationship with the psychiatrist but feels himself powerless to change it:

No, I'm not happy with it. Dr Perkins hasn't the time. You wait one and a quarter to one and three-quarter hours, and you're in three minutes and out. 'Come back in twelve weeks!' There's no explanation given why they've changed these drugs, he just rung for the nurse who brought the prescription through, he signed it, she took it back and I went, and they put it into me. They didn't say, 'Right we're going to try a brand new drug on you, we don't know the side-effects', they didn't say anything like that. I mean, I might be a guinea-pig, I don't know. It could be a brand new drug, or the combination could be brand new, mixing this drug with what I already have in me.... I'd like him to explain what were happening.

Has he ever told you about the illness you have had?

No, he does the talking.

Have you ever asked him?

He doesn't reply. He's superior. When you walk in, you sit down.... Between you and me, he's superior to me, I'm the patient and he's the doctor.... *He* does the talking.... I wish he would spend a little bit more time and explain, explain what the side-effects are going to be.

Harold, who has been receiving treatment for almost twenty years, describes his relationship with doctors in similar terms:

I'm used to answering questions and not asking them.... The only time I tried to question my doctor was when he was going to give me electric treatment. I asked him what he was going to do with the electric treatment. At the time he told me he was trying to channel my thoughts.

Nevertheless on occasions he has been able to negotiate with doctors over his medication:

At times I have objected to something, and I think they've listened to me. For instance the injection I have is Modecate, once a week. Before that I was on Haldol and it was causing me problems. I told them about it and they eventually stopped it and put me on Modecate.

Even when patients are informed about side-effects they can be given very partial accounts. So, for example, Rachel apparently believes that tardive dyskinesia is only associated with high dosages and does not appreciate that it often occurs when medication is stopped:

When they first gave me an injection I had a very bad side-effect when I was in hospital. Apart from that I haven't had any side-effects – I'm hoping that tardive dyskinesia is not for me. . . . It's apparently something that if you're on high dosages for long periods you might get it – but I've been told that there's no sign of that at all that I might even be beginning with it, so that's put my mind at rest from the point of view of side-effects. That's the only side-effect that seems to be mentioned.

Another, and perhaps, stronger version of the battle with the doctor which many people describe is given by Sarah. In Sarah's experience of mental health professionals, people with a history of severe mental illness are always at risk of being patronised and so have to fight for recognition, to get people to accept 'Look, my mind's as good as yours or as strong as yours!' Sarah is insistent that she can make her own responsible choices about her life.

You're having an old battle with your doctor – 'I want to come off my medication!' 'Oh, if you do you'll become ill again'. You have to be really strong, you have to say 'Look maybe I won't become ill again'. Then it's a personal choice of yours but you have to really go back to them and say: 'Look, I want to come off it'. I'm going through it at the moment. While you're on medication you're always going to be sleepy or ill or not perform like you used to be able to perform. So that's the next stage I'm going through with my doctors, trying to get off the medication.
The idea of becoming ill again, what does that do to you?
It's frightening, but to me I have accepted that, OK, I may be ill again. Therefore I'll take the risk and be prepared to do it myself. Of course they say: 'You'll become ill and you'll cost the NHS a lot of money'. The nurses say that, not the doctors.
What do you feel if they say that?
It knocks your confidence back again. You have got to be really sure of yourself and a strong person and be able to say 'I'll risk it'.

She goes on to say

If you accept medication *you* have to go away and live with it. . . . They don't know what they are giving you. You have to go away and cope with the sense of feeling tired and all the rest of it. They have never experienced that. All they know is that it stops the schizophrenia from happening but they don't know the side-effects and all the rest of it and how else it affects you. It's all right the doctor giving it to me but I'm the one who is taking it and its up to me whether I should take it or not in the end.

Lastly we come to Ben. Ben sees himself as having a mental illness but he thinks of it as precipitated by stress:

> I have got a mental illness, I wouldn't contest that I haven't, but I believe it's stress related and sleep related rather than genetic or chemical.
> So if you are talking to a psychiatrist is that something you are likely to discuss with him?
> Yes.
> And what action do you think they would take?
> I don't think they would take any notice.... I believe that their heads are full of chemistry and my head is full of politics and social things. So that's a conflict that perhaps won't ever be resolved.

He feels put under pressure to take medication for his illness:

> I have a family – my brother-in-law is a doctor and my sister is a nurse – and people around say 'Look lad, you have to take your medicine' and so the power and authority of the hospital medics I can't do anything about. I just have to take it. There is nothing I can do about it. I just pray that they will get it right.

Nevertheless when asked whether he feels the medication benefits him Ben replies: 'Yes, I feel it is doing me good'. It was then put to Ben that in the light of his own experience the medical view would seem to be backed up by evidence. Ben's rejoinder to this is interesting and summarises what to a large extent is a shared perspective among our participants on the failure of medical authorities adequately to address the psychosocial dimensions of the predicaments of people with a history of mental illness. 'Yes', he says

> but it's not the *only* thing. ... I think this is where the problem comes in. A doctor treats *a patient* and he looks at it, he's patient-orientated and my contention is that I get mentally ill because of social problems. I will take a good instance, my mother was in hospital and tried to commit suicide – my father in my opinion was the mentally ill one because of his behaviour but he never went into hospital. Now they never solved that problem because

they never tackled my father. And in the same way, although they tackle me and give me these injections and so on, it will continue to happen because of the social problems involved. Do you see what I mean? If you like, I am the symptom of something outside, the cause is outside, whereas they would see the cause as me and if they solved me, solved my problem, then everybody else is all right. And so it's an eternal conflict!

CONCLUSION

We shall discuss the implications of this exploration in more detail later but perhaps the most consistent message that comes through here is that in participants' experience of services the significant questions that concerned them about the value and direction of their lives were left unaddressed or obscured. Medication was judged to be beneficial but delivered crudely, as the primary form of intervention, it became a currency that devalued participants' efforts to re-establish their personhood and resist entrapment in an unremitting state of mental patienthood. For the most part services appeared to offer participants a form of protective containment within the identity of a community mental patient. As our participants saw it, such containment did not generally provide a means or stepping-stone to a more meaningful form of inclusion in social life as much as confirmation of their own marginalisation and lack of social worth. An image that was often borne upon us when participants discussed their experiences of services was of containment in a confined space cut off from where they and others judged the significant action to be. Most of all, agents wanted purposive activity that, as Barry expressed it, appeared to be leading somewhere. Only then could they be said to be doing something more than 'passing the day' or 'filling their time'.

3

ON THE EDGE OF
THE COMMON

INTRODUCTION

For many of the people we are concerned with the transition from
ordinary living to mental illness and its consequences was abrupt and
shocking. Sarah described how she felt as though she had been
'kidnapped', and Simon that his life 'just came down like a pack of cards
. . . it was a shambles suddenly, almost overnight'. However, brief
though the journey may be in one direction, the road back is long and
arduous. As we have seen, our participants found themselves in a
precarious predicament in social life in which they experience difficulty
in securing trust and respect as ordinary human beings and in
establishing a reliable material foundation to their lives.

From a theoretical point of view there are three distinct ways of
conceptualising this type of predicament: as a *transitional* state through
which people move on their return journey to an achieved and settled
form of personhood; as an *occasional* state to which people who have
made the journey back to an achieved form of personhood periodically
return; and as a *continuous* predicament or struggle within which we can
detect variations and possibilities for movement but which those who
find themselves in it cannot properly be said to leave. With one
exception it is this last category which most adequately identifies the
type of predicament in which our participants found themselves and in
this chapter and the next we shall explore some of the variations in the
continuity of their struggles.

'IS THE ILLNESS BEHIND YOU?'

To mark the contrast we may start with the one person who had edged
beyond the predicament of the displaced majority into an achieved and
reasonably settled form of personhood. This was Anne, a woman in her

70

early forties who had first broken down in her late teens and during the ensuing years had spent long periods on a refractory ward for chronic schizophrenics and when out of hospital had lived rough, sleeping in parks. From being a 'rubbish-bag lady' Anne has progressed through numerous upheavals and false starts to a career as a nurse in a general hospital. Generally speaking, she feels she can hold her own alongside her colleagues, but at certain critical moments the knowledge of her psychiatric past is brought to the fore:

> There was a staff nurse that came, and she didn't know that I had been ill, and they were talking in the office one morning and I got very angry because they had asked me to do something, and they were all sat down, so I blew my top and said why couldn't one of them do it . . . and I stormed off into the back room, and I was really mad, and this staff nurse came in and someone must have said something to her and she said 'I wasn't getting at you, Anne' and I said 'Nobody said you were getting at me, I didn't think you were', and I just said 'Go away, go away', and after that she said she didn't know I had been ill, and she didn't really know how to treat me sometimes, because if I got mad I think I frightened her, and she didn't know quite how to treat it.
>
> Did the other people seem a little bit on tenterhooks because they didn't know whether you were just angry or ill?
>
> Yes, quite a few times.
>
> What would they do then, did they run round helping you or did they withdraw and leave you to your own devices?
>
> Well, there used to be one girl there called Sandra and she always saw the funny side of everything, and when I used to get mad she used to try not to laugh but she used to laugh and say 'Anne is having one of her do's' and so she used to see the funny side of it.

Anne can be said to have re-established her personhood but at times like this she can be reminded that personhood is not a tenured accomplishment and that in the eyes of others it can very easily once again be put in question. She is aware that in order to sustain her identity as a capable person, her vulnerability can only be very partially acknowledged and that she must manage her stress as best she can off-stage in her own time. She recognises that there is always the risk that it might declare itself on stage and that she would then, in effect, have forfeited her lines:

> Do you feel the illness is behind you now?

71

Not completely, no, because from time to time I do get ill. Even with the injection, if I am under a lot of pressure and worry, and then I am real tired, then it comes on. But not very often.

Does that worry you in any way? Does it mean it is always in the back of your mind?

I just sort of think when it comes on, well it's here again, a couple of days rest and I'll be all right and it will pass.

So you do literally take a couple of days' rest?

Well I just usually hope it's my days off and then rest and it recedes.

What would you do if you felt it coming on now for example, would you just say 'Well I have got to work tomorrow and the days after I can rest'?

Well, I'd go to work tomorrow and hope I'd rest the days after. But I don't know what I'd do if it came on properly as I wouldn't know what to say.

FORCED INTO THE WILDERNESS

In the remainder of this chapter we shall describe the experiences of seven people who within the field of social and cultural forces we have identified have difficulty in establishing a satisfactory stance for themselves in social life and find themselves on the fringes of what we may think of as a common life. In looking at these various experiences of estrangement it should not be supposed that we are attempting a classification of the characteristics of individuals. While we shall certainly be dealing with instances where the effects of the illness is particularly severe, there is reason to suppose that the chain of causality involves a number of factors and it would be misleading to assimilate outcomes to the effects of the illness itself. It may be more helpful to think of these experiences as variants within a common struggle, as examples of a shared structural predicament at its point of maximum severity. Clearly the characteristics of individual agents are a factor here, but so are chance and circumstance and agents who are presently unanchored and demoralised might well, if their circumstances were adjusted and the options open to them extended, prove themselves more viable strategists in the conduct of their lives.

Where Anne has succeeded in establishing a responsible role for herself in a busy and demanding institutional domain, in Melvin's case the force of his own disturbance periodically propels him to abandon structures of human association altogether and to take to the woods and

72

moors. Melvin is a man in his early fifties who first started to experience severe symptoms, such as voices threatening him, ideas of being possessed by evil spirits and observed by the Special Branch, some twelve years ago at a time, it would appear, when his marriage was in jeopardy. He was last in employment as a labourer on a building site some four years ago but was forced to give the job up because the voices were distracting him. Voices and disturbing ideas continue to trouble him and to interfere with his everyday business and he describes how, for example, he sometimes finds himself leaving his bag and goods behind in the middle of the supermarket because he feels that the Special Branch are monitoring him. Until recently he lived in a self-care hostel but over the past two years when the voices became unduly pressing he frequently left the hostel for the neighbouring woods and moors to try to find some respite for himself, sleeping rough for two or three days at a time, and wearing plenty of clothes to keep himself warm, 'a big coat that comes down to my ankles':

> I started wandering off, kipping out because the voices were telling me to get out. I just kipped in the woods.

On occasions Melvin has also broken windows in order to get himself put into prison and the safety of an environment where he felt the voices were less likely to trouble him. But as soon as he was put away he could hear the voices telling him that they were pursuing him and he came to the view that the woods and moors would afford him more protection because he would be able to spot the voices coming to get him. To start with the strategy was successful and he had quite a few weeks of tranquillity both on the moors and when he returned home, but the periods of respite became shorter and shorter and eventually disappeared altogether:

> The last time the voices were with me when I were camping out and with me when I got back.

Like Harold, Melvin sees himself as engaged in a war with the voices. He explains how they ease off when he leaves the house because 'they've won the battle sort of thing, and got me out of the house, that's what they want'. He now feels that he should, perhaps, not have capitulated and that if he had stuck it out and stayed at home he might have fared rather better.

When we last saw him, Melvin was in hospital having, in effect, been admitted from the moors. In contrast to the image that one might perhaps have of him he was quite smartly dressed, with worn clothes but a tie and polished shoes. He did not want to stay in hospital but nor did he want to return to the hostel and he had just been allocated a ground-floor council flat in a high-rise block. The aspect of his life that meant most to him was his tenuous but much-valued connection with his family. Of his four children he has always managed to maintain contact with the eldest and he also spoke with special pride of the youngest, the 'brainy' one at grammar school. His own active life he saw as being behind him: 'I can't do anything now, I'm tied down, you know, with my illness.' None the less he was looking forward to moving into his new flat, and getting furniture for it with an allowance that a social worker had acquired for him. He appeared to suggest that after years of moving from one form of temporary accommodation to another since the breakdown of his marriage and the onset of his illness he now wanted to settle down. As to whether in his new situation he will still feel driven to take himself off to the moors is, of course, quite another question.

'SECOND-CLASS CITIZENS'

Henry and Sally are two people for whom the marginalisation and isolation of ex-mental patients in social life, and the low regard in which they are held by others, had come to be accepted as facts of life, unamenable to change. As we described in Chapter 2, Henry is an unemployed man in his late thirties who feels humiliated by his living situation in a ground-floor council flat on a run-down estate on the outskirts of the town. Shame over his social predicament troubles him much more than his illness:

> The voices haven't come back. I'm pretty stable there because of the Modecate but you just feel ashamed at being unemployed so that when people ask me am I working I don't like to tell the truth. I just walk away because I'm ashamed.

Looking ahead:

> The future is grim. I find it hard to work, I have always found it hard to work. Everyday I have bad feelings if I'm on the go. I get a lot of tension and depression and anxiety and other feelings I don't understand anyway. As long as I keep getting these feelings I feel a fear of people, especially in the working situation and if I get these feelings I will never be able to work. But the injection does help to take the voices away. I was thinking of witchcraft

74

and Jesus Christ and all sorts. It was a dreadful illness. That's gone now but there's nothing else the doctors can do for you apart from give you Modecate and look after you in hospital for a while.

When he thinks about his life uppermost in his mind is the feeling that

I would like a job and would like to live a normal life without schizophrenia. But that is not possible and never will be. I have always had ill feelings throughout my life which make me feel upset and depressed because I am going to have tense and anxious feelings.

What he is most in need of is company:

I need to go somewhere where people are friendly and I can talk to. I have been to the YMCA and like to go somewhere where there is someone I can talk to, but people don't come up to you and talk to you. You just sit there reading a magazine.

Yet Henry does have one close friend whom he met in hospital:

When I first met Kathy in the hospital she was suffering from depression and we went to the pub and she said she has been in and out of hospital – she is about forty years old – we went to this pub at about Christmas last year, that's when I met her. She said 'What made you poorly?' I said, 'I might tell you one day when I know you better', and she said, 'Did you think you were Jesus Christ?' As I said, she has been in hospital and seen a lot of mentally ill people, so how she guessed me being Jesus Christ I don't really know!

Kathy has a relationship with another man but over the past year she and Henry have developed a close friendship:

I think she likes my company. That's it, I think we just like each other's company. She gets depressed and she just needs a sympathetic ear and she knows that I have a sympathetic ear so I never drag her down and she feels safe with me and I feel safe with her.

The other compensating feature in Henry's life is his car for which he saved £4 a week over nine months from his Invalidity Benefit. It is, as he describes, a 'gamble' but

them wheels make me feel better. It gives me a bit of security because I can just go from *A* to *B*. When I am really fed up at home I can just go out. I do feel more adequate because I have a car.

Nevertheless his overall sense of what life holds for him is bleak:

> With schizophrenia you are not living, you are just existing. There is not a lot of future for you, but you come to terms with the illness. I don't like telling anybody but I do accept it. I am labelled for the rest of my life. . . . I think schizophrenia will always make me a second-class citizen. I go for an interview for a job and the anxiety builds up. . . . I haven't got a future. It's just a matter of waiting for old age and death.

Sally is a year or two younger than Henry, has had several admissions to hospital and lives on her own in a council flat. She says of herself:

> I'd like to be married but when you're a psychiatric patient, when you've had all this illness, it's very difficult to meet anybody. I don't have any social life, so how can I meet anybody? . . . . I get so depressed because I sometimes feel as though I have no future. I just think I'm going to be a psychiatric patient for the rest of my life with no social life and not much money and I don't see any future for myself.
>
> Do you think of yourself as a psychiatric patient?
>
> I do, yes. I do, yes.
>
> In what way, because to be awkward you're living here in a flat, you're not in hospital?
>
> No, I'm not, but I still need the hospital. I need to ring them up, I need to talk to the nurses and the doctors . . . and I still need to take all my tablets – I take a lot of tablets. I don't know, I just feel as though I am, you know, a psychiatric patient.
>
> And what does that mean, being a psychiatric patient?
>
> Well you just don't feel the same as everybody else, like I say if I wanted to meet anybody I'd feel as though I'd have to almost apologise for my illness, to try and explain my illness. To try and be accepted, that's it. It's as though you've got to try and be accepted by people, to be normal, you know, to say 'Look I'm normal, I'm normal, but I've had all this illness'. . . . It's like you've got to try and make people understand that you are normal, you know.
>
> What about here on the estate? Do you know any of your neighbours here?

No . . . well there's Mrs Jones downstairs and she's lovely. She's in her eighties and she's a really nice lady and I talk to her sometimes.

Do you talk to her about your situation?

Yes. I think Mrs Jones doesn't think I'm odd or anything. She knows about my illness and she always asks me how I am and that. You see, unless I tell them nobody would really know that I've had all this illness. But it's like when you want to make a relationship with anybody. . . . You think, well what do they *really* think? Do they think I'm mentally ill or what, when you tell people, you know?

Sally plainly feels that she suffers from a vulnerability for which she stands in continuing need of medication and contact with psychiatric services, but it is at the same time apparent that her self-ascription as a psychiatric patient comes from a different set of pressures. The statement 'I feel I'm a psychiatric patient' functions here not as a description of what she actually is, or of a role to which she has been assigned, but as a negative definition of what she feels about herself as a person and of the life prospects that she judges to be available to her.

In Henry's usage 'schizophrenia' is not so much the name for an illness as for a social predicament to which the experience of illness has given rise. For Henry coming to 'accept' the illness and coming to 'accept' an impoverished conception of what he can reasonably do and hope for – of his significance and value – have been brought to merge in a painful experience of exclusion and worthlessness. In what they say about themselves Henry and Sally illustrate not the *natural* consequences of mental illness, but the *social* consequences of becoming mentally ill in society as they enter into the person's most intimate sense of who he or she now is. We can, perhaps, think of these as examples of how under the kinds of pressures we have described a man and a woman may be brought to think of themselves. It is not by his illness that Henry feels crippled – by his own account it is now to a large extent under control – but by the social pressures and constraints that have turned him into a person devoid of worth and prospect.

'WAITING FOR THE ELECTRICITY'

Henry had at least his car, and Sally a satisfactory housing situation, but the predicament of Bill illustrates a more desperate form of disconnection from social life, exemplified more concretely by the fact that he has been waiting for almost four years to have the electricity connected in his home. Bill is 39 but could be taken for 59. He had his first breakdown when he was 26 and has had a number of periods in hospital, the longest lasting three years. For the past four years he has been living on his own with a dog in a council flat on a large, run-down post-war housing estate on the margins of the town where he has been allocated one of what are unofficially recognised as the 'hard-to-let' properties most prone to vandalism. The flat is extremely neglected, all the windows are broken, there is no electricity or gas, no furniture apart from a sideboard, a battered settee and a mattress, no sheets or blankets, no cooking facilities of any kind – Bill eats out of tins – and the floor is covered in dirt and dog excrement. It was a sunny day when one of us visited but the air inside the flat smelt dank. The wallpaper was discoloured and spotted with black mould, peeling off the walls in several places, and in others held on with sellotape.

For three years Bill was a patient in a large mental hospital, one of the old county asylums, just across the moor from the town where he used to live. Bill liked it there – he worked in the hospital gardens for which he received £12 a week, and felt himself to be relatively well off. Of an evening he would often walk across the moor to the town:

> I'd see my mates, go for a pint with them, then walk back down to the hospital, get my tea, go down to the Red Lion at night. There'd be a group of us would go, we used to go out in groups.

Bill didn't too much mind being a patient in a mental hospital. Generally the staff didn't bother him much and he was left to go his own way. He looks back without resentment on the altercations he sometimes had:

> I used to have a do with old Fred now and again, he'd put me in lock-up. I'd go crazy with him, and start shouting and bawling at him. He'd get on top of me like [laughs] and we'd have rows. And he'd put me in lock-up and give me a needle to quieten me down. He'd leave me in lock-up for about an hour or two while I cooled down.

Bill would have been happy to stay in the hospital but after three years

> They got me a flat. They decided I was all right and I could look after myself, or try to look after myself, rather than be hospitalised all my life. So they got me a flat in the town and I was doing all right there until I stopped going for needles and they stopped

coming to give me needles. They said I had to go up the hospital for them. Well I didn't go. Why should I go to them when they should come to me? So I did without them and had another breakdown then.

Bill then spent a year in another different mental hospital and after that a social worker found him his present flat in an urban environment a considerable distance from the town where most of his friends still live. Resettlement in the community has thus entailed, for Bill, a significant form of displacement from his actual roots in community. It would be misleading to overstate the strength of these roots but they did represent such social connections as he had. From Bill's point of view, certainly, the mental hospital in which he spent three years was an 'ideal environment' in that it both provided him with a condition of dependability and also permitted him to retain his connections in the world outside. Over the past four years he has lost contact with most of the people he knew and now leads an extremely isolated life. Even allowing for some exaggeration (as we learn later, Bill can still find the price of a pint), his memories of the amenities that the hospital afforded him throw his present situation into grim relief:

> There is nurses there to look after you all the time. Better facilities there than I have here – you can watch television and listen to the radio, go for walks round the grounds, go for a pint at night which I can't afford to do whilst I am paying rent for this place. I can't afford to go out – only with the dog. If I were in there I could go for a drink, I could afford to smoke a lot more than I am doing at the moment. . . . They've got washing facilities, like washing machines and spin dryers, and you can go for a bath at any time you want, there's always hot water, plenty of hot water. . . . I was getting three meals a day which I am not doing now and am surviving mostly on sandwiches till I get my electric on. This past four winters I have gone through hell, having no gas and electric.

One of the windows to the flat has been boarded up by the council because Bill broke it himself and couldn't afford to pay for the repairs. When Bill moved in, the gas was connected but he fell behind with the bills and the supply was cut off. However, he has been waiting four years to have his electricity connected. Some months ago he received a visit from the electricity board. The man

> checked the wiring with a little meter thing and he said it's not

safe to turn on. He went over to council office so I had two days waiting for a fellow from council to come. He come with a meter and he said he'd be back after holidays. So after his holidays he come, he had his little meter, he unscrewed all the plugs and the sockets, he said 'Oh, we can't turn it on, it'll have to be all rewired. Try turning it on it'd blow place up!' So I've been waiting for them. I'm still waiting!

He has been waiting for three weeks and hasn't been able to go anywhere:

It's depressing stopping in looking at four walls or sitting outside waiting for them. I've been sitting on wall at end here so I can keep an eye on the flat for when they come.

He describes how he manages to survive in his situation:

I seem to get through all right. Like this week, I haven't done so bad. I mean I've got plenty of dog meat as you can see. I've got plenty of cigarettes, I've even got plenty of biscuits in. I saved up for a four-pack of coke. I had a four-pack yesterday, and that's me second loaf of bread.
Is dog meat the first thing you buy?
Yes. Always think of dog first!
Just take today, for instance, what have you had to eat?
Fish and chips, beef sandwich and chocolate biscuits.

Bill's hardship is aggravated in the winter:

Funnily enough this is the worst winter I've known. It's been cold this winter, I really felt it. I had to go and beg some blankets which I wouldn't do normally, I make do with what I've got, overcoats and that. But I had to go and beg some blankets from advice centre. They gave me a couple of blankets up there.
How did you feel about that?
I felt embarrassed.

After he was discharged from hospital in 1983 he was brought to the flat by a social worker:

What happened then?
The social worker – she were a good lass but she went to work somewhere else so she lost touch and I haven't been in touch with anybody since then.

So no one has actually gone out of their way to get in touch with you?

No.

And you haven't got in touch with them? You haven't tried phoning or anything like that?

No.

Is that because you feel it's not worthwhile or do you just feel you don't want any contact with them?

I don't really want to bother. I'm trying to live by myself and get out of relying on people. I mean, same as going back to when my father were alive and he died in 1964, and left me working in the mill looking after my mother and four kids. Now I was working then – I was working three nights overtime and Saturday morning. All my money was going to my mother to keep us all. Mind you I bought my own clothes, she gave me enough for my clothes and stuff, overalls, everything like that.

Bill's mother died in 1969 and at that point

everything seemed to go wrong. The mill closed down so I were out of a job. The family broke up. My youngest sister went to live in Ireland with relations over there, me and my youngest brother we went to live at Y, my next brother in line he went to live at F and got a job down pit. And my youngest brother, he got a job in the supermarket filling shelves. And I was lucky then because he was able to get me a job as a warehouse manager. Then he packed up there and went to work at a paper mill. And I packed up and went on the dustbins. From dustbins I went on to roadsweeping. From roadsweeping I went on the rubbish wagon. Now the best job I had were that on rubbish wagon because we used to go round country cleaning cesspits out for farmers.

But eventually he was made redundant:

So I packed it in altogether. I went up to Scotland for a while. My brother come up and talked me into coming back. And when I were up in Scotland I were out of work then. I was living in a tent at the bottom of Ben Nevis, near Fort William. I was only getting £6 a week, that were me dole money, with not having a fixed address like. I had to go and sign on every day, but even then it left me plenty of time for wandering round the mountainside and that, looking at different plants and animals and birds. So me brother came up and talked me into coming back

81

down, and that's when me troubles started then, trying to find a job.

Bill eventually had a breakdown in 1973. Shortly afterwards, three of his four brothers got married:

> and only one asked me to the wedding. Because of me going into hospital, said I were loony like, you know, mental. They didn't want to know me any more. Only one of them, our Jim, he invited me to his wedding, he come and got me out of hospital for the day.

Now that he has been back in hospital again none of his brothers will have anything more to do with him:

> It were all right when I were making a go of it but when I ended up back in hospital they all lost touch then. So the only contact I've got with family now is my sister.

Bill is happiest when he is in the country and most of all would like a job on a farm. He often goes on long walks for about twenty-five miles with his dog, starting out when it gets light, and generally goes to bed as soon as it gets dark. His sister lives not very far away and Bill visits her every week or so and takes a bath there but, according to Bill, her husband doesn't like him to call more often. He gets his benefit on a Thursday and in the evening meets up with a friend:

> When Sam were out of work we used to meet at dinner time on a Thursday every fortnight, because he got his giro fortnightly. So we used to arrange to meet and have a game of pool. We'd listen to records and talk. . . . Then he got this job and he goes down on a Thursday night now. So I changed me pattern from Thursday dinner time to Thursday night. It's that every week now. It's better. We're drinking on a Thursday night, we have a game of pool, a few games of pool, a few pints, then fish shop, a couple of chicken legs, and home.

Bill likes being solitary, and doesn't really want more social contacts, but nevertheless

> I keep looking out for an old girl-friend when I go down by canal. I keep hoping I'll see her down there, I haven't seen her for twenty years. She's probably married now and got a family.

He has recently started missing his injections again but knows that he will have to go for the next one because his sick note is due and he won't be given another one unless he attends:

Missing one or two you don't notice it, but if you go a long time then pressures build up, till it's like now where I'm getting behind again, I've got behind with my rent again. I get so far behind, you just go crazy, trying to make ends meet again.

He says that he could very easily have another breakdown:

I start hearing voices, start imagining things, people coming to the door, people banging on the door. Neighbours get on your nerves, banging, walking across the ceiling.
    Can you actually hear them or is that part of your imagination?
    Well, you can hear them but it plays on your mind.
    Can you tell when there's a breakdown coming on?
    You have an idea and it's time to go to hospital then and see a doctor.

When things start to go wrong:

It sounds strange really. You start feeling like committing suicide, doing daft things. . . . I tried to hang myself once but the neighbours stopped me, told me to ring the hospital up, so I did do. I got in touch with the charge nurse I know and she told me to come straight up to the hospital, not to bother going back to the flat, just get on bus and straight to the hospital. As soon as I got to hospital she got an emergency doctor to me and they kept me in for three weeks.
    When you said you tried to do that, was it because you felt low and miserable and fed up, or was it because you perhaps heard voices telling you to do that?
    Partly that I heard voices, but I know that I were miserable, I were depressed, because I had nothing to do. Winter time it was, and it were cold and damp, and I didn't even have dog then. It's not so bad with dog, at least dog gets me out. Especially now she's on heat!

Bill has little or no hopes for the future:

Not really. As long as I die in peace, no pain. . . . My father was only 38 when he died. He died of pulmonary thrombosis. He'd come in from work, he'd been on nights. . . . He was an

83

overlooker in a spinning mill. My mother was 42 when she died, so there's not much chance of me going much further.

Since the mental hospital told him that it was time that he learned to look after himself, Bill has been left to fend for himself in a predicament in which all his significant connections – with friends and acquaintances, with psychiatric support services, with the material supports and connections that are commonly taken for granted – have been all but severed. There are redeeming features to his situation – the proximity of his sister, his relationship with his dog, the friend with whom he drinks – but it is hardly surprising that his thoughts should sometimes turn to the mental hospital as a preferable alternative to the terms of existence in social life that have been offered him. There are certainly ambiguities in Bill's stance. The disconnections he experiences have very largely been imposed upon him but it is also evident that he prides himself on his ability to go it alone and 'get out of relying on people'. Yet for all his defiance, continue to rely on other people he recognises he sometimes must and it is noteworthy that he possesses a keen sense of the liabilities in himself and is willing to resume the connection with psychiatric services – to visit the doctor, phone the hospital – when he judges it necessary.

'DOING WITHOUT SERVICES'

Terence and William are two people exceptional in our participant group in eschewing self-recognition as suffering from a mental illness that requires treatment, despite both their histories of hospitalisation. Terence is a 34-year-old Irishman who, since coming to university, has lived in England for the last ten years. Since leaving university he has had a number of hospitalisations, spent time in prison, wandered the country and slept rough for a period, and lived in a Salvation Army hostel. Despite his psychiatric history he is reluctant to admit to illness, preferring to ascribe his behaviour to other factors such as anger. Here, for example, in describing his difficulty in conveying anger without acquiring the diagnosis of mental illness, he hints at an implicit Irish racism that manifests in the increased likelihood of psychiatric labelling:

> I used to get very angry and I found out that it's 'Not On' (affecting an English accent], it just doesn't work to get very angry in England.
> Is that because you're Irish?
> Yeah. You're going against yourself if you get angry. You've

got to be a different sort of person altogether to get angry and get
away with it you know. . . . You've got to be English born and
bred to be angry and successful at it.

Later he touches on this again when he is asked about how he feels
about being labelled:

I can't always feel angry about it because that would be leading
them [the doctors] back into mental illness again.

Though he denies that he has been mentally ill, none the less the
shadow of 'schizophrenia' hangs over him:

I came across a book with the word 'schizophrenic' in it. It was a
book on mental illness and I was terrified that this might happen
to me. I was even terrified when I saw the word because I
thought I might be that. . . . I knew what it was and I looked to
the Freudian definition of schizophrenia as a split personality, so
anytime I came across that in my own personality I would sort of
'join together' and say: 'No, I'm not!'

Implicitly he acknowledges that he has had schizophrenic experiences:

As far as I'm concerned I really wish they'd leave people alone
who hear voices and have visions and all the wonderful things or
nightmare things that can happen to schizophrenics. . . . If
anybody asked me I would just say, 'If someone wants to be a
schizophrenic and wants to see visions and hear voices and
everything, then let them just do it.' I'd just say, 'Let them alone
. . . as long as they've got somewhere to live.'

Terence has no friends, no contact with services and appears to want to
be left alone to pursue his solitary course. Yet it is also evident that his
isolation pains him:

There's only certain people I can talk to. If you imagine yourself
in a position like a goldfish where you're among people that you
really cannot talk to very much at all, only on a superficial level I
mean.

Though he claims to want to be left alone, he is also at points equivocal:

I suppose it's people that disturb me more than anything. I don't
really disturb myself. If I was left alone in this room, just dreaming
at night, I could live quite happily. . . . But then I *do* want to
make friends as well.

By virtue of his education Terence feels an affinity with the professional classes but his experience of the medical profession appears only to have heightened his sense of isolation:

> Doctors don't often understand you. My doctor in the rehab unit used to shut me up. He wouldn't let me talk at all. He didn't *want* me to talk at all.

What seems to worry him most is the idea that in the popular understanding of them labels like schizophrenia set the people to whom they are attached apart from their fellow men:

> My experience, and talking to other people that have been in mental hospitals ... obviously some are tortured and disturbed, but so are lots of ordinary people. In fact the line between when you are in a mental hospital, rehabilitation hostel, the line between yourself and an ordinary person is very similar – the only thing is the stigma attached to your being there, so you can't get a job. That's what it always comes down to, not getting a job.

Terence is still without a job but he does now have somewhere to live that he finds satisfactory. Until recently he had been living in a Salvation Army hostel and spending the days either wandering the streets or attending a day shelter, but the worker at the shelter has now helped to find him a place in a self-care hostel. The move has clearly made a difference to his sense of himself:

> You sound very optimistic now, more so than when I last saw you, when you were at the day shelter.
>   Yes, well I do. Everybody wants a certain amount of comfort and somewhere to live that's decent. So when that happens you feel you're progressing.

Having a room of his own at last is important:

> And food! You can eat when you want to. You can go to your room when you want to. You can buy records.

Though his material circumstances have improved, Terence continues to feel isolated and uncertain. He intends to struggle on without recourse to psychiatric services, and at times feels that his chances are as good as anybody else's as long as his psychiatric history doesn't catch up with him. But he experiences also great difficulty in accounting for the collapse of his life-project over the past ten years and in assembling some sense of worth and prospect in the face of a history of failure:

86

I get this sense of . . . almost as if you've come down a little in the world. Is that accurate?

Yes, I have, and that is the most difficult thing to come to terms with. I don't think I've come to terms with it yet, but at least I find the answers more easily. I don't find them as difficult as before.

His current situation, he goes on to say, 'doesn't really square with my idea of myself – nor with the reflection of my idea of myself that I get from my family'. For example he no longer holds out much hope of getting married:

I might never get married.

Why's that?

Because I might never be given the opportunity to get married. I don't know – I want a job first of all, but I don't know. I want a career or whatever, but I'm confused about that. . . . I would just say that I want a job, but *I* know what *I* mean by that, I don't want any kind of a job. . . . I might be unemployed for the rest of my life. . . . I'm 34 years old now and I've had just about enough of life. . . . I can't go any further. . . . I just want to get a job, get married and get on with getting a home of my own like a normal person.

It is not clear what answers Terence now gives himself, but it is plain that they are not answers that help lead him out of his isolation. We can sense in Terence not only a fear of failure but also the additional fear that if he acknowledges mental illness he will be crippled still further, irretrievably lost, that he will find in psychiatric treatment not a means to understand what has happened to him and a resource for dealing with it in some measure, but only a hideous confirmation of his only failings.

William is 40, he has suffered from mental illness on-and-off for the past twenty-three years, and last had a job eleven years ago. The following is a brief acount of William's history over the past ten years. In 1978 he was living in a bed-sit in a run-down area of town where he started to feel increasingly depressed and vulnerable. According to William, people were constantly 'banging on the windows', his 'so-called friends' proved to be no good, and William became more and more isolated from what few people he knew.

In 1979 he was recommended for rehousing on medical grounds and was allocated a 'hard-to-let' flat on a housing estate on the periphery of the town, but two years later after constant problems with his neighbours he again made an application to move. In 1981 he was transferred to another flat on a nearby housing estate. Again, he suffered the problem of 'noisy neighbours' and made many complaints to the council. In 1983 he was allocated another flat half a mile away. Here he was broken into twice and had to contend with drunks and 'sinister' noises from the neighbours at night, and children name-calling and throwing stones during the day. Again, William complained to the council. In 1987 William moved to his present address, a sixth-floor inner-city flat, where he lives alone with his parrot and cat in three rooms. When we came to know him he had been there six months and he was, he said, starting to experience problems with neighbours 'banging on the ceiling'.

William has no friends and though he says he would like people to talk to, he rarely goes out because he feels looked down on and finds it difficult to mix. His only social contact is a sister whom he sees very infrequently and he expects, for example, to spend Christmas on his own. He occasionally goes into town and wanders around but he hates the place – 'You're better off on Mars' – and spends a lot of time in bed. He has left the town only once in the past two years – on an outing to the seaside from the day centre which he attends once a week. In principle he would, he says, quite like to spend more time each week at the day centre but not if it was a question of 'just sitting around'. He watches a lot of television, and plays games on a microcomputer which he acquired on hire purchase, but he often feels fed up and depressed and sometimes contemplates suicide. He sees a GP from time to time but refuses to take the medication that is prescribed for him. He recognises that people treat him differently because of his solitary behaviour but he doesn't see himself as 'mental' or as schizophrenic.

Someone like William is, perhaps, easily prone to think that the people who live around him are intentionally molesting him, but as his housing saga brings out he has been forced to live in conditions in which he is indeed very likely to be molested. Interestingly Terence appreciates the kind of difficulty that William experiences in his council flat:

> There is a problem if I was envisaging myself living in a council flat. The problem would be other people around me and the social problem there. That would kind of filter into my brain. I'd start thinking 'Are there vandals there?', this sort of thing . . . I think you've got to keep to yourself if you move into one of those flats, you've got to cut yourself off.

Terence and William have certainly been made to suffer the socially ordained fate of the isolated ex-mental patient, but in their case it is perhaps a fate which they have also exacerbated. William and Terence both very much keep themselves to themselves and cut themselves off. They both see the self-ascription 'mental illness' as a capitulation or humiliation and as a consequence they suffer doubly – they suffer all the ravages of isolation and exclusion, and the depletion of self-respect, common to many ex-mental patients, without the help of a framework to make sense of what has happened to them and the solidarity that comes from sharing with others in a similar predicament.

GETTING A BREAK

Harold's life is normally led within the confines of the structural isolation in which the other participants described in this chapter found themselves. But here we shall illustrate how even a relatively minor event can make a significant difference, and permit the re-emergence of buried sources in someone who generally characterises himself as a 'loner'. In many ways Harold appears to be self-sufficient, makes few demands on social services and, apart from seeming a bit withdrawn, outwardly displays little or no sign of what anyone would define as 'illness'. However, all is not well as aspects of his illness, combined with unremitting poverty, lack of social contacts and poor future prospects mean that his life is a continuing uphill struggle. What, among other things, Harold stands in need of is an occasional holiday but lack of resources and diffidence in social relationships mean that people like Harold rarely have the opportunity to permit themselves a break. Generally the only break Harold gets is on admission to hospital for the odd day or weekend when the pressure becomes too much for him:

> I don't get a break at any time, I've hardly had any breaks at all actually. . . . Now I've got another year upon me [this was his birthday] . . . I don't think I'm going to get a break this year either, really, from the household chores and things, unless I go into hospital . . . and then I really won't get a break there because I have to do things there as well.

Last year, though, Harold did get a proper break because he managed to save up enough over four months to take part in a trip organised by two social workers in their free time. One of the social workers reported that Harold was a different person on holiday, much more talkative, and from Harold's own account it seems that he discovered in himself a potential that belied his description of himself as a loner. When he spoke to us about his experience we had never seen him so animated:

I had to save to get the money. A quid a week for quite a while. It cost £20 for five days. We had a minibus, we travelled around, had a good time. There were two social workers from the district and a couple of care assistants. We went to the Dales, Morecambe and the Lake District . . . and went down the pub.

What was the best thing about it?

Oh, the release, the pressure being off. Just getting out and away.

How frequently have you been out of Northtown in the last three years?

Not more than twice a year.

How did you get on with all the people you went with?

Oh, we got on all right.

You said to me that you like to be on your own, that you're a solitary type.

I didn't mean it that way, I didn't mean that I was a loner as far as times like that was concerned, oh no, I mix in. I mix in here as well. I mean, it's like, I've no woman, I haven't managed to get one, I haven't had the health to get one. As far as close friends go, most of them are now married. Any that I had in the past, they're all married as far as I know. So I don't mix with any of them any more.

You said that getting away was a big release. It sounded as if when you were away you were living quite close together with people.

Yeah, it was all right. We had to share the cooking, washing. . . . We had a coal fire, one guy had to carry the coal, one had to keep the fire going . . . we all mixed in together, we all got on well.

If you had the opportunity would you like to go again?

Oh yes.

4

BATTLING ON

REASSESSMENT AND 'ACCEPTANCE'

In this chapter we shall explore some of the ways in which people with
a history of schizophrenic illness develop an understanding of themselves
and their situations over time, and learn from hard experience to
become active strategists in the reconstitution and negotiation of their
lives. As we have seen, a severe schizophrenic breakdown typically
wreaks havoc upon the agent's sense of his own biographical continuity
and telos, upon the narrative coherence of his life. To start with it may
not seem that there is much the agent can do to control his fate. For
example Bob was asked what advice he would give to a younger person
who was experiencing a schizophrenic breakdown for the first time:

> I don't think there is any advice you can give except that you've
> got to find your own destiny through it. . . . I used to feel like a
> pin-ball in a pin-ball machine being banged about all the corners
> and the bumpers and things like that. You actually feel like that
> when you're having a nervous breakdown. . . . You're out of
> control. . . . The ball has to find its own way out of the pin-ball
> machine somehow.

But there comes a later stage where the person may be brought to
recognise that he needs to take an active stand and attempt to take hold
of his destiny. For example Simon described how his breakdown

> buggered me life up completely, that's for sure, as it has done for
> so many people that I've met. It completely throws a spanner in
> the works. All me plans, I mean I was doing well at college and I
> was going to go on to a degree course theoretically, I'd even
> applied to the sorting thing for the degree, and it all just came

91

down like a pack of cards. . . . It was just a shambles suddenly, almost overnight.

Simon in many ways epitomises a form of moral progress from devastation through to the recognition that something has to be done. For more than a decade after his first breakdown it seemed, as he put it, that 'nothing was happening' in his life, there was no sense of *movement*. He no longer felt himself to be an agent with a life to live. Over this period he was admitted to hospital on numerous occasions and desperate to cut loose from a condition of constant mental patienthood he eventually decided to take what seemed to him the shortest and most direct route back to ordinary living and to do without hospitals and treatment altogether. To start with he succeeded and managed to secure himself a job as a clerk, but he had not reckoned with the liabilities in himself, and as a result

> I ended up going back to square one, sort of thing, well *worse* than square one . . . I was sectioned.

The shock of this reversal brought about a change in Simon. He came to judge that if he was to reconstitute himself as a person who was not defined by his history of illness and to recapture some of the ground that he had lost, then he had to accept some measure of responsibility for his aggressive tendencies. Looking back over the history of his difficulties he recognised that aggression had for some time been an expression of his disturbance:

> I got very aggressive, not at first but pretty quickly I got very aggressive with people. I started to swear at people in the street, spit in their direction sort of thing. I became quite poorly with it all really, in fact that's why I ended up getting on section eventually. . . . About three years ago I thumped an old guy in the street. I got stupid with it, I just knocked him down. Fortunately I didn't do him any harm but that's not to say that I couldn't have done, and I got put on section. Fortunately I don't react that way any more. Occasionally if I'm feeling really angry I'll swear mentally but I don't spit and kick and hit people or anything like that any more.

After he was admitted to hospital on section:

> the one thing I were absolutely certain about was that I wanted to get the hell out of there, so I just started – the drugs didn't do me

any good, they just made me feel poorly – what I did was to sort of mentally tell myself over and over again that I must control me anger if for no other reason than the immediate reason that I'd get put in isolation if I started hitting people. . . . So the very first thing is that you had to control your anger in the hospital, and then I knew that long-term I had to control me anger anyway when I got out of hospital otherwise I'd be back in again. And through gradually learning to control me angry feelings, it worked out that I gained control of myself, if you like. I started to work me own problems out, I suppose you could say.

Sidney describes a similar experience of actively attempting to fight his illness:

Is it something you actually *do*, or do you just allow yourself to get better?
I don't think I allow myself to get better without a little help. You really have to fight it to bring yourself back to reality.
What sort of form does that fight take?
Like I say, in my illness I have a tendency to daydream and misinterpret ordinary events, and they seem to have special significance. I have to think very carefully whether I'm behaving rationally myself.
I see, it's like monitoring your every thought.
Monitoring, yes that's it.
That's hard work is it?
It is when you're not too good to start with.

Over the past three years since he was sectioned Simon has decided that 'rather than just let the status quo exist' he has got to 'change things and start improving things'. An essential condition of change for Simon is breaking free from the psychiatric system:

I am determined that if there's any chance at all I'm going to clear the system, get off benefits and get some sort of work and something meaningful.

However, the experience of his last reversal has taught him that there is no short road to the goal that he has set himself. For three years now he has managed to stay out of hospital but during this time as well as learning to bring his aggressive tendencies under control he has also, as we described in the last chapter, decided to make cautious use of official psychiatric settings. Simon recognises that this is not the road he actually wants to travel and that if he does not keep his wits about him it could prove to be a dead-end, but he has come to see it as a useful means of testing himself out for the next stage of his journey. He has learned from experience that he cannot assume that all his troubles are behind him and that there are forces in him that he must reckon with and assimilate into his understanding of what he is and can do:

> You just have to accept that you've got these problems and you've just got to cope with them as best you can and keep your patience and hope that you're able to cope.... One of the reasons for going to the North Road Centre is that I'm going to have to now for five days put up with people full-time. Now if I can do that successfully – and I've had no trouble today – I'm pretty sure I can do, but if I make absolutely certain, and do it for any length of time, then I know that with a college course or a job there's a very distinct chance I'll succeed.... It's like doing it in stages, isn't it ... North Road isn't like a job in a lot of senses but I've never found work any problem, it was always people that were a problem, and therefore North Road should be just as much a problem in theory as a job. Mind you, convincing an employer that that's the case, that's another thing!

He is keenly aware of the uncertainty of the road ahead:

> It may be that given a college course for two years that I'll do the same, just a repeat performance of before, I'll stick it for so long and then suddenly find again problems. But I'm pretty sure, as sure as I can be, that that isn't going to be the case.

Simon recognises that for someone in his predicament to be sure as he can be is by no means as sure as he would wish. Although he now *feels* more hopeful about the future, he sometimes worries about the *grounds* for his hopes:

> I think it's reasonable because I've gone quite a while now without having to go back into hospital. I've gone about three years since I were in there and I've never felt that there's even the slightest chance of going back in there, I've never deteriorated and I don't think I've ever gone that length of time before becoming poorly. So I think in *that* sense I'm pretty hopeful. It's just that you always know that you've got to be realistic and that whatever you do you could end up back to square one.... But there's no point in saying 'Oh, I'm going to end up at square one

so I'm not going to even try'. You've got to give it a try and see
what happens, haven't you?

The threat of reversal to 'square one', as he terms it, always hangs over
him:

It takes away some of your confidence. . . . You know full well
that the odds are stacked against you and that people are going to
be less tolerant of you than somebody else who's had no problems
in the past. It knocks your self-confidence and makes you sort of
think, 'Well, I *hope* this is going to be so' whereas somebody else
would say, 'This probably *will* be so', because there's no reason
why it shouldn't be. You know there *is* some reason why it
possibly won't be, and so it takes your self-confidence away – to a
degree, not totally, but to a degree it takes some of your
confidence away.

Like Simon, Sidney is cautiously trying to rebuild his life and he helps
us understand the sorts of dilemmas that people in his predicament
confront and the quite complex assessments they have to make:

Do you see yourself getting back to work at some time in the
future, bearing in mind the unemployment situation here?
   I'm fairly hopeful, I'm quite confident that I'm capable of
getting back to work, but I've no incentive to. I regret that I'm
dependent on the Social Security, I'd like to feel that I was
earning my own keep. The shameful thing about it is . . . I'm too
well off. For the time being it'll be best. . . . I've no financial
incentives to go to work. I can cope quite well with what money
I've got. The incentive to work would be to mix socially. I find
that very difficult. I'm frightened of it because it might make me
ill. That's a minus, not a plus. What I need is to feel *useful* and
there's not a lot of jobs that can offer that.
   Does that enable you to plan for the future then?
   I still don't trust myself really, to go out and get a job and start
being a bit ambitious, I daren't. I feel that that could lead to me
becoming ill.

By most people's standards Sidney would not be considered 'well-off',
but he does at least have the security of a steady income from the DHSS
and he can be reasonably sure of things carrying on the same way one
week after the next. Were he to apply for a job, on the other hand, his
guaranteed benefits – including housing benefit – would cease, with no

95

certainly that he would be able to sustain the job for very long. He might then find himself in the difficult position of having to go through the complex procedures of negotiating a new claim for benefits when not in the best of health. From Sidney's point of view, therefore, getting a job is a high-risk undertaking that at the present time he does not feel it sensible to pursue.

BATTLING ON

No matter what skills people may develop, they always have to contend with the emotional wear and tear of battling on, and sustaining optimism, against innumerable obstacles. All of our participants seemed at some point to have succumbed to the bleak sense of 'acceptance' to which Henry, for example, has been brought. It is difficult for a person to remain rationally optimistic in the face of so many difficulties and set-backs, and it is perhaps the case that the more people with a history of severe mental illness learn about what is at stake for people like themselves in our society the more ungrounded their optimism must become. Hence we can, perhaps, understand why Bob in the space of a few minutes should give two rather different accounts of how he sees the future:

> Really I want to make myself a home somewhere and settle down and have a reasonable place to live – whether it's a council place or private I'm not bothered. . . . Find myself a place to live so I can settle down and feel comfortable in my own house or flat, find a job with the help of some study at college, and just take it from there. . . . I'm *reasonably* optimistic in the sense that I feel I can do that now.

But then a little later the future looks rather different:

> I try not to think about it too much. I'm not very optimistic. The only bright light is that I can do some studies at the Polytechnic and then I'll soon be eligible for Community Programme jobs, so I can apply for those. . . . I'm more optimistic than I was immediately after my breakdown, I thought I'd never work again, but I can't say I'm very optimistic actually.

Yet many of our participants managed to hang on to a sense of their own life projects, to the romance of their lives, in the teeth of what had happened to them. For people in these predicaments to keep going requires a good deal of self-knowledge, together with experience of the social and cultural pitfalls as Simon described so well. And it requires also courage. Many of our participants complained about their isolation and wanted more social contacts but most of them envisaged living out their lives on their own. A number of people had been married in the past (Bob most recently to a nurse whom he had met in hospital), and Sarah was uncertain about her prospects, but only Vaughan seriously entertained remarrying. The rest were either doubtful about whether their circumstances would bring them into contact with the right person or, like Ian, judged that they could no longer handle a marital relationship.

We can learn from Sarah what is involved in trying to sustain an optimistic sense of one's life project and to resist the bleak sense of 'acceptance'. Now in her mid-twenties Sarah had a severe schizophrenic breakdown not long after completing a degree at university and subsequently spent a year in hospital. She described the shock of mental illness and its consequences, the radical displacement in the community of her life, in the following terms:

> It's just like being kidnapped. . . . The world stopped for a whole
> year . . . not doing anything, and I couldn't account for it.

When she left hospital she felt 'better' but she quickly found that there was no easy return passage from mental patienthood to living an ordinary life. The enormity of her loss, and the challenge to recover it, was daunting:

> You've got to build yourself up again from nothing. From being
> right down at the bottom you've got to build yourself up again.

The task, as she saw it, was nothing less than to start 'establishing' herself 'as a person' all over again. As she felt, the only way to confront her predicament was to embrace the challenge:

> I've just got to accept it. I've got to say 'I must like it when the
> chips are down'. You've got to say it. You *don't* like it, but
> you've got to say it. It's like a defence. You've got to say, 'Oh, I
> like it when the chips are down'.

She feels that the illness has brought about

> A definite change in me. It's a change, a definite change, I
> experience.
> Do you think you could get back to how you used to be?
> No.

97

That was someone else was it?

Yes, maybe one day I'll be able to go back to being a *similar* person, but not the same person.

Generally speaking we have a clear idea of . . .

Who we are, yes. Well if you're a schizophrenic or whatever you have to fight more for your own individuality. You lose your individuality, you completely lose it. You sort of merge with other people and listen to their ideas, get their ideas into your head and you just lose yourself completely. Because you haven't got that barrier in your head which says 'I disagree with you, I'm going to say this'. You haven't got that in your head any more.

Sarah says that she no longer has

the same emotions and the same feelings that I used to have. I haven't got the same control over my emotions that I used to have. . . . Emotionally you feel like a star that's just exploded, that's how you feel.

And now?

Half in between the two. Sometimes I feel all right, sometimes I don't. Sometimes I go right back to the beginning and sometimes it's all right.

Yet despite the changes in her, and her abiding sense of vulnerability, Sarah refuses to permit her identity to be defined by her illness:

My fight, my personal fight, would be to say: 'No, it's not going to affect the rest of my life', and that's why I struggle so much, because I don't want this illness. I don't particularly cherish it or want it or go on about it as if it were the bee's knees. I'd rather be normal.

As we have seen, the person who had a severe mental illness is always a questionable person, a person whose status is open to radical doubt. As Sarah recognises, there are different ways of responding to this experience of being put in question. Sarah's response is to attempt to resist the force of the question and to challenge the cultural and social obstacles that are put in her way. She accepts that she has had an illness, and that she continues to be vulnerable, but she will not allow that she must therefore live in permanent exile from ordinary personhood. She goes on to distinguish her own combative stance from the ironic embrace of the 'professional nutter':

That's just me. Like a lot of people react in a different way.

There's one I know who says, 'I'm going to be a professional nutter for the rest of my life, and he laughs about it, and is able to joke about it, and that's his way of accepting it. But I can't do that. . . . I've never accepted it, I don't think I've ever accepted it.

BACK TO 'SQUARE ONE'?

People carry on in the knowledge that for every advance there is the possibility of a reversal. The shadow of another breakdown hung over all our participants and the metaphor of a return to 'square one' was commonly used. For many people it was clearly important to attempt to devise ways of moderating the impact of a set-back. The question that people asked themselves was: must having a relapse demolish everything, such that the person has once again to confront the shambles of his or her life? This was a matter about which people felt deeply, and sometimes said contradictory things. Vaughan brings out some of the difficulties that are involved here. He now has a girl-friend with whom he is tentatively planning a future and who appears not to be influenced by the negative images of schizophrenic illness which vitiated his relationship with his former wife:

Before I was fighting the wife and the children because they were all against me, but now I have somebody on my side, so it is a lot better.

When he was asked how he saw the future Vaughan said:

Well I know that by 10 October I am out of a job. As far as the illness goes I am trying to get a full-time job but I might be out of it again. I'm definitely going to end up back in the hospital in the next three years.

Is that a bit daunting and does it frighten you at all?

No, I'm used to it, I've been in there twice. I look on it now as just a way of making new friends, meeting new people.

You're working at the moment, you've got a girl-friend, you're planning for the future, you're saving, you're doing all that, but you know something awful is going to happen to you which might undermine all your plans and yet they are still going ahead?

Yes, I'm still going ahead but I have to talk it out with my girl-friend. She says she's not bothered if I have to go back into hospital from time to time. It's just . . . well, I met one woman – she had two children – and she was telling me the doctor says

'Every six months you have to go back in hospital', and she doesn't see the children. You've just got to accept it.

As we shall see Vaughan was not always as buoyant about his capacity to withstand disruption as this, but on this occasion he attempts to moderate the impact of what he takes to be an inevitable set-back by assimilating it into a relatively optimistic sense of himself as a viable person. After such a reversal, he goes on to say, he will find himself further back down the road than he is now, but he believes he can recover – in six to nine months on his own assessment – the ground he has lost. His benignly opportunistic view of what a spell in hospital affords him may be considered a rationalisation, but it is certainly one way of assimilating what might otherwise be experienced as a dismal reversal into the continuity of a life-project.

One of the concerns shared by many participants was that they would once again find themselves homeless after another breakdown. It is here, perhaps, that the experience of a return to 'square one' registers most forcibly. In Vaughan's case, for example, the house in which he had been living remained empty for the four months he was in hospital and as a result it had been broken into, his possessions stolen and his flat set fire to. Vaughan had nowhere to go and found himself in effect abruptly discharged to the street. From his account of what the doctor said to him it appears that the doctor viewed 'getting better' as a circumscribed medical event in which the personal and material disruption that the experience of illness brought in its train were not accorded much significance:

> I saw the doctor on the Monday and he said 'You're going home on Wednesday'. I said I had nowhere to go and he said, 'Well, there's nothing I can do, you're better now and you can go home'. So I was a bit bitter then, I thought I was just getting kicked out and nowhere to go.

At the doctor's behest Vaughan duly left the hospital for the streets on the Wednesday but as it happened was lucky enough in the next few days to meet another discharged patient from the hospital who had already managed to secure a flat and was looking for someone to share. But others, as we have seen, are not so lucky. From his own previous experience of homelessness following admission to hospital, Barry is also alert to these consequences and is anxious to insure against a repetition. Like Vaughan he accepts that his illness is likely to recur in the future and having recently moved into a housing association flat his main concern is to ensure that he can hold on to his home as a secure place to return to if he has to be readmitted to hospital.

A number of our participants also described how they had learned from their first experience of illness such that the second time round they were able to involve themselves more actively in their own treatment, and to moderate the disruption that would otherwise have ensued. So, for example, Bob describes how

> the second time I realised I was ill. I didn't know what was wrong with me but I realised I was ill. . . . That enabled me to cope, realising that I'd been through something like this before, it enabled me to cope . . . to realise that I would get better therefore, you know 'just hang on in there'. And it took me much less time to get over that than it did the first one.

On the first occasion, by contrast, he was a passive and bewildered recipient of medical attention:

> I had no idea what was happening to me, no idea at all, even when they were pumping me full of drugs. . . . I was very withdrawn then, I'd been staying with my parents for ages, I'd been out of work and all I did all day was read, eat, go to bed, sleep and that was it. I wouldn't talk to anybody. I was very withdrawn. Presumably I'd been slipping into this state for some time. . . . I was hearing voices and I had all those weird experiences, but I had no word to describe them then, I didn't realise there was anything wrong with me.

Though he does not relish the prospect, Bob now feels himself to be better equipped to deal with the prospect of a breakdown than he was in his teens. Having a breakdown, he says, is 'like going through a black hole in space':

> I think if you have a major breakdown like that, when you've come out of it, at the other end of it, outside the other end of the black hole or whatever, you feel psychologically stronger and more mature. So I think if there was an 18-year-old lad, and he had a breakdown like that, I'd feel very sorry for him because I don't think he'd have the maturity to cope with it very well. It would probably take him longer to get out of it than it would me now. I don't think I will ever have another breakdown like my first one.

He hopes that his illness is now behind him but

101

Occasionally, like this weekend . . . all I can describe is I feel very strange for a bit. What I do is just lie on the bed or go to sleep or try and get through the day with it, and it's usually over by the next day, but it lasted for a couple of days this weekend. . . . To all extents and purposes I just try and relax as much as possible and say to myself 'I've been through bad times before and it'll pass' and it does pass.

But the 'bad times' don't always pass and there comes a point where people may take it upon themselves to negotiate a potential crisis and seek out professional help. As we saw in the last chapter, for example, Bill felt able to visit the doctor or phone the hospital when things were becoming too difficult for him. However, it became apparent that in attempting to negotiate a crisis the person may not always be able to convince psychiatric experts that he is as knowledgeable about his inner states as he claims. Sidney, for example, knew that he was 'becoming very ill' and that he could no longer cope on his own:

> The last time I went into hospital I actually got there the previous night and asked to be admitted because I was aware I was ill, I knew things weren't right with my family and that. . . . The next day I had more or less a total breakdown.
> Did they admit you that night?
> I couldn't convince them that I was mentally ill.
> Did anyone take any notice of you that night?
> My father was very sceptical . . . I couldn't really . . . I had no one to talk to.

As Sidney went on to describe, he knew in himself that he was becoming 'more and more out of control', but because at this point in time he was not behaving in the way that a person with an acute schizophrenic illness is supposed to behave in order to merit ascription as such, the hospital sent him on his way with the rebuff that his mind was merely 'fantasising'.

A HAPPINESS IN MADNESS?

The reassessment of a life in the face of a mental illness involves difficult questions, not least in the appraisal of the experience of personal upheaval itself and what it implies for the revaluation (and in consequence often devaluation) of the person. In the first of two

excerpts from a group discussion between Ben, Frank, Sarah and
Vaughan we highlight some of the tensions and ambiguities that may
arise here. So, for example, the tension between an experience of
devaluation and a process of revaluation in which people struggle to find
point in what has happened to them and what they have become;
between a grieving for lost opportunities and a lost expression of
selfhood, and the discovery of value, across all the complications of their
lives, in the sorts of people they have turned out to be. The experiences
of personal upheaval are variously described as funny and exciting, or as
traumatic and hellish. For Ben and Vaughan they have been traumatic as
much as exciting but where Ben hankers after an artistic potential in his
own turbulence that he has felt himself unable to express, Vaughan
desires only the tranquillity of a garden. The assessments people make
for themselves may also at points be at odds with the norms by which
people who are prone to these sorts of experience in our culture are
expected to think of themselves. In this excerpt one of us starts by
asking, which have people found the most difficult to cope with, the
illness itself or its consequences?

Sarah:	I'm guilty of enjoying my schizophrenic experience! [much laughter]
Frank:	I agree with you. If the psychiatrist said to me, 'Look, Frank, we're going to give you a tablet and we're going to make you normal when you've taken these tablets', I'd be very uncertain as to whether to bloody well take it or not, I'd be frightened of what normality would mean to me again, actually, after such a long time. I think I should be frightened of it, quite frankly.
P.B.:	Why?
Frank:	Well, looking out at the majority of people that are considered normal and then looking out at the kind of happiness I enjoy within my illness – I think I'm a damn sight better off than the majority of those people, I do!
P.B.:	The happiness you enjoy within your illness, can you say . . . ?
Frank:	Yes, that satisfies me. I don't demand a lot in life.
P.B.:	You're nodding at that, Sarah.
Sarah:	You're poor in a lot of ways – OK you haven't got a car and you haven't got a house – but you're a damn sight better off in a lot of other ways. Not *better* off,

not better off, but you are reasonably content most of
the time in your illness.

Frank:　There's a happiness that comes with madness. . . . No
way would I take a sanity pill again, no, no!

P.B.:　You said just now, Sarah, that you're guilty of
enjoying your schizophrenia. Can you say more about
that?

Sarah:　Well, what I should have said really is that I was
happier being schizophrenic, and having all these
thoughts and all these things, than what I am now –
going through life and trying to cope with the
normality of life. I'm not really guilty of it, but to the
doctors I was a pain in the arse and to everyone else I
was a pain in the arse – that's why I've come to say
I've been guilty of enjoying it!

P.B.:　So in a way the whole notion of it being an illness has
to do with the trouble it caused other people – is that
right?

Sarah:　To other people I had to be locked away and all the
rest of it. If they'd left me on my own I'd have been
perfectly happy. . . . When it first started I went to the
doctor with the idea that I could be cured. Now I've
realised that that's a load of baloney – you're not ever
cured, you just have to learn to accept it and live with
it. So I made the mistake when I first had it, I went
straightaway to a doctor and said 'Look this is what's
happening', and they took me into the hospital. And
after that it was tablets and things to stop it but while I
was going through it I really enjoyed it. I've never
been so happy as what I was then – I've always got
that to remember. . . . Not just because you've got no
responsibilities or anything, it's just all the thoughts
you're having in your head, it's like reaching a peak.

Ben:　I agree with you, you know. I believe it's some kind
of experience you have which is difficult to explain –
it can be funny, it can be traumatic – but it is an
experience that if you were an actor, if you were on
the stage or something, portraying it, you wouldn't at
all be . . . you'd be . . . or a creative artist actually
putting it on the paper or writing it down . . . but it
actually happens in your head, and you can perceive it.

Frank: And all the world's a stage. . . !

P.B.:   So for you, schizophrenia wasn't painful then, Ben?

Ben: No, it has been horrible as well.

Vaughan: I had some hellish experiences but also some where I was as high as a kite. They were great, but the other ones, they were out of this world. . . . I think that's the only time you end up in hospital – when you're having the pleasure side of it you're not bothered about hospital.

P.B.:   But what about Sarah then?

Sarah: I knew something had happened and that's why I went in. I sort of panicked, I wasn't able to cope with it by myself, so that's why I went in. While I was in – I don't know, to start off with it was really bad and then I got into hospital, and it became really exciting and I went through it. . . . And then towards the end it was getting bad again and that's when they decided to stop it and they gave me more tablets and injections. So it's like a mixed experience.

R.H.:   Was it an experience that you wanted to end?

Sarah: Not at the time. At the time I'd have carried it on, I'd have carried it on.

Vaughan: Yes, but my experience is that you're feeling really good and high, you're getting all these thoughts and you're the happiest person in the world – but in my experience after that comes the hellish thoughts and that's the only time it gets me. . . . When I come down it goes the other way and that's where all the problems start . . . I mean, no one wants to change it when you're high, do you, it's brilliant!

Sarah: Except when your parents are coming in to see you all the time, and you see that they're upset and all the rest of it, that's what makes you think 'Oh well, there's something wrong, something *different* about me'. That's the only thing that sort of brings you down to reality again – the fact that your parents are coming in and crying and all the rest of it. Otherwise, when you're having it, you're perfectly happy aren't you?

Vaughan: You must be different from me. I've got good memories of the hospital from when I was going through a bad patch.

Sarah: The only bad memories I've got is the way the doctors diagnosed me and treated me, that's the only bad side of it, the way they'd come up say 'We're going to do this to you' or 'We're going to do that to you', whereas really I didn't want anything – I just wanted to be left to carry on.

P.B.:   I suppose the question arises from what you say – why do you see all this as an illness? In terms of your description of the experiences, why then classify it as an illness?

Sarah: Because I know that I have the vision of waking up one day and feeling all right and the next day waking up, and I thought 'Something has happened and I've changed inside'. That's why I class it as an illness – that's the only way I can remember it and that's the only way that I can say that it *is* an illness. . . . That's being perfectly honest.

Ben: I think if I had the ability to write down my experiences or paint them, I wouldn't be a famous artist but people might think 'Oh, that's interesting, that's an interesting view' . . .

Vaughan: Yes, but would anyone believe you? I mean, some of mine, if I told you mine, you wouldn't believe me – well, maybe *you* would but not anyone who hadn't had them – they were just so weird and bizarre. You wouldn't believe them unless you'd experienced something like that yourself. It were true to life when it happened but I couldn't explain it to someone. . . . In my experience, once you start getting these hellish trips you don't want to live, you just want to commit suicide. You don't want to put it down on a canvas, you don't want to put it down on anything!

Ben: Well, I know but you're not an artist and it's not what
          . . .

Vaughan: I just want a garden!

'MAKING IT ACCEPTABLE TO YOURSELF'

The second extract from the group discussion illustrates several of the issues we have discussed, variations in Sarah's phrase on the theme of making it 'acceptable to yourself'. As we have seen, prior to this sequence the group had been in a lighter mood and identified some of the gains they had derived from their history of mental illness, in part despite the experience of pain and displacement, in part through that very experience. Yet on balance they would all rather have done without it:

Ben: I would rather have been without it.

Sarah: I think so, yes.

Frank: Depending on what normality would have meant to me in the first place, I wouldn't want to go through it again. I've spent two-thirds of my life locked up in hospitals and various other institutions for practically thirty years so I think that I can categorically say 'Definitely not, no!'

Vaughan: No, I don't think I could go through it again. I sometimes regret going through it in the first place. . . . I just want to, well I don't expect too much now, I just want things to keep on as they are really. I think that's my own fear – my one big fear – is of having to go through it again and it coming out again . . . and having to go through all that. . . . I wouldn't say it were an advantage going through it!

Sarah: When you've been through it, you have to learn and you have to adapt.

Vaughan: Oh yes.

Sarah: It's something that happens and you have to make it acceptable to yourself. You have to accept that a lot of things that you might have been doing you can't do anymore, and things like that, you have to learn.

Frank: You have to learn to conform to the limitations which you come to know of your own life . . . and I think in the end that you learn to accept them. In the beginning, perhaps, you fight against them but you do come to accept them.

Vaughan: One thing about it is that you do get a few warning signs when you're going to become ill . . . sometimes you can just feel, 'Well, it's coming on again', and you nip up to the hospital and tell the doctor.

Sarah: But I don't think any more like I used to, 'Oh it might come within a week or it might come within a month.' I've been on a level now for about two years so the fear of it coming back again is gradually receding.

Vaughan: Yes, that's it, you're sort of living in fear of it coming on again, aren't you? I think that's your worst problem.

Sarah: But so what? If it does, it does – you just have to accept it and you just have to go through it again.

Vaughan: Yes, but what you've built up while you've been on the level.

Sarah: So it crashes down and you build it up again, don't you!

Vaughan: Yes, you've got to start again.... But every time it gets a bit harder doesn't it? I've suffered twice or three times, it's got a bit harder each time.

Sarah: But at least you know what you're expecting ...

Vaughan: What you're expecting, yes.

Sarah: That would be the advantage of it. You know when you go into a hospital what it's going to be like. That would be the main thing.

R.H.: What is the difficulty – is that you've had the carpet taken from under your feet and you have to start again, or is it your confidence that's taken a knock?

Vaughan: Yes, your body and your spirit, it all ... your mind, body and soul takes a knock.

R.H.: I can see how materially you may go back to square one – and lose your job or your flat. Is it also an equivalent knock spiritually? How do you get over that – is it something you let time heal or do you have to grit your teeth and start to decide very determinedly to march forward and start doing something new?

Vaughan: I found it quite impossible to do anything. You sort of lay back and let it pass and ride the storm. And then when you're feeling a bit better, then you can start. But it takes time.

P.B.: You were smiling, Sarah, when Bob said 'grit your teeth'?

Sarah: Well it's a question of.... You have to throw out a lot of ideas that you used to have when you were ill. You have to make a determined effort to throw out those ideas and I think you have to be twice as strong mentally to cope with what you've got to go through.

108

P.B.:   Can you give me an example of the kind of idea that you have to throw out?

Sarah: Well, when you go through an experience you get all sorts of ideas into your head – that people are all connected or something like that and you have to really make an effort to throw those ideas out. For instance, now when I talk I always wonder whether it's coming from me as I used to be or whether it's coming partly from schizophrenia. . . . I think you do have to throw out a lot of ideas . . . [pause] . . . It's the only way you become well again.

Ben: I think I would agree with that. You kind of reassess your life. I was determined to get myself integrated into society in some way because I felt out of it. . . . So I joined various groups and things – things that I could cope with. . . . The opportunity of employment was pretty grim but I'm now employed and I'm quite happy . . . well, for a year anyway. . . . In some ways I'm not satisfied with what I'm doing because I was quite ambitious really and there were things that I wasn't able to do. So really I've gone backwards.

Sarah: Yes, when it first starts you sort of fall down – you've got all these ideas, all these plans of what you want to do, and they just crumble . . . and then you have to start again.

R.H.:   It's hopes and aspirations that are taken from you, perhaps, is that it?

Vaughan: Yes, I think I lost all my ambitions. I just sort of took it from day-to-day, not expecting too much.

R.H.:   Is it a kind of narrowing of people's horizons, would that be true?

Ben: Well, it's a kind of acceptance. In some ways for me it's an acceptance of failure, and also an acceptance of a continuation of failure, because I feel that I couldn't do that much without socially being stigmatised – people saying 'You've had a mental illness, you can't cope with this job' or 'We won't let you cope with it' . . . So there's a kind of failure and an acceptance that I won't be able to do those things. . . . So that's the first thing. Also some of my aspirations are down and I simply look for simple achievements – getting a job and getting an increase in wages and things ... small achievements, really.

Sarah: Why don't you do what you set out to do – is it because you feel less confident in yourself or something like that?

Ben: In some ways I've ... there's a reaction, I feel I don't ... I don't feel I could really cope with some high-pressure job ... and that I know my place! [laughs]

Vaughan: Yes, I had my heart set on being a driver. I paid so much for these driving lessons and passed my test. Once I were in a car, I had no problems and I thought 'That's it, I'll get a job driving, no problem!' But things didn't work out. It doesn't bother me now.

Ben: I feel that I just have to accept a society which I don't really agree with – the vast amount of great wealth and things, and a social system that encourages greed ... I look for simple things, friendships and things.

Vaughan: I think that's important – friendship. I think that's number one priority.

5

REVALUATIONS

CREATING AND SUSTAINING VALUE

Largely because they are so often forced to live in exile from the kinds of valued roles that alone among our participants Anne now occupies, perhaps one of the most difficult problems for people with a history of severe mental illness in our society is to sustain a sense of value. One way to attempt to combat the menace of devaluation is through the giving of accounts that aim to redress the 'official' view of the person's history as the story of a wasted life. So, for example, Steve endeavours to furnish a narrative of his life that highlights his accomplishments as a painter and decorator who until very recently always managed through years of illness to get back into work after he came out of hospital. Though he still does a number of odd jobs on the side, he now feels his age and assesses that with his injections he could no longer manage a full-time job but in the past

> You see, I were always good at climbing, I could get up a sixty-foot ladder, that's why I always kept me job.

In providing an account of himself as a resourceful and hard-working citizen, Steve endeavours to counter popular attributions of the person who has suffered from schizophrenia as 'dishonest', 'lazy' and 'incompetent':

> I know that I am mentally ill and that I need treatment, but me mother always swears that it's not schizophrenia. You see, circumstances alter lives don't they? I mean, since I've come out of hospital I've had no trouble, well I've never had any trouble with the police in me life because if I want something I'll work for it and if I haven't got it I'll do without. I'm not a thief, I wouldn't con or rob anybody. I used to do jobs all the time when

I were married, I'd be working nearly every weekend for myself, and I've done jobs round here. . . . I can't walk down the village without somebody saying 'Are you still doing jobs?' Because whereas I'd get £2 at work, I'd charge them £2.50 at weekends and it were tax-free in me hand and I did a bloody good job.

Value in the struggle

The following examples illustrate the lives of two people who under conditions of considerable hardship and isolation have both turned the challenge of their solitary life-projects into a strong focus of value and learned to derive a sense of pride from their achievements in maintaining the struggle. Philip is 45, lives on his own in a council house, and has managed to stay out of hospital for ten years. He views acute relapse as a form of surrender which he has learned to resist: 'Now I don't go through the door any more and capitulate'. None the less he still suffers from what he describes as a form of 'nervous debility' in which 'you feel as though you're burning all over'. It is as though, he continues, 'you had a cut on your hand and someone was always fiddling with it, and making it bleed. Your nerves are totally raw'. Only if the ex-mental patient becomes *hardened* to stress, he says, can he expect to survive in society. Becoming 'hardened' involves, as he puts it:

An acceptance of your fate in a way. You've either got to accept that position or go screaming crazy.

He recounts how

I have managed to survive for ten whole years and it's a hell of a long time when you're suffering quite a bit. . . . I wouldn't recommend it to anyone that term of existence, it's been hell really over the ten years, but when you're at the bottom of the pile there's the old saying beggars can't be choosers and that could apply to my case.

The rigours of what he feels he has to contend with become no lighter:

Well, you asked the question what does the future hold out. Quite honestly just sometimes I feel very suicidal, I don't think the future holds much at all. . . . I'm now 45 and when you can go for – since this problem first started, virtually my whole life

I've been under some strain ... and when you can go forty-odd years and nothing much happens to improve your lot, I mean you're virtually in the last third of your life and nothing has been done. ... There might be a motive in ignoring people with illnesses. I hope that the illness will go away but *they* hope that the person having the illness will go away! ... It's terrible really. It's really negative all this stuff but really that's how it is. ... What you do look forward to are the occasional times when you don't feel quite as bad as you did. ... I do feel better on occasions and I don't know why this is.

Philip complains that he has to manage on his own with little or no external support but for almost ten years he has to a large extent kept himself to himself and made little or no effort to make his needs known to official agencies. During this period he has been prescribed minor tranquillisers by his GP but he has received no anti-psychotic medication:

The fewer drugs I take, the better I feel. ... You're able to function as a normal human being as far as possible.

He recognises the contradiction in his own stance:

I said I hadn't seen anyone for ten years. ... I was saying earlier that I should be seen every month but I haven't been anywhere to see anyone for ten years! It seems crazy doesn't it! You see, I'd rather keep myself quiet. It's the pride business – if I can manage I will do even if I feel terrible. I often think when I get my mental powers back that it's not a bad thing to be in here ... I have a certain pride, I have a certain pride, in trying to cope with whatever is wrong with me.

Moreover his experience of psychiatric functionaries has not been encouraging:

I have little regard for psychiatrists. I've had bad experiences with psychiatrists and nurses, so I don't get in touch with people. They really do give you a punch in the guts. For instance, I said I was suicidal to a nurse and she said 'Why don't you do it then?'

Philip particularly prides himself on maintaining his house in impeccable order:

It's part of survival. I can actually see a worth of being here. I can

113

make a difference to something, affect something ... I feel as though I've accomplished something.

The person with a history of mental illness, he says, always has to struggle with the feeling of 'worthlessness'. Philip tries to maintain his sense of worth largely through his passionate interest in railways – he is an active member of a local railway group, and has three thousand photographs, which he took himself, of rolling stock – and through a local history project on which he has been working for a number of years and which he sometimes doubts that he will ever complete. Philip feels that his mental powers come and go, and that at points he is much worse than at others. He describes how he copes with his 'nervous debility':

> I think you cope with it by regimenting the way as to how you live. You organise your week on a certain basic pattern, and you follow that pattern virtually every week of the year. And, funnily enough, it has its advantages, but also its disadvantages, because if something goes wrong with the regimentation, or the pattern, you start to panic a bit and if you can't carry through that method that you have organised for yourself, you think that you're sinking, that the ship's sinking ... That's a metaphor, really, for saying that your health's not quite as good as it was, and if your health isn't too good you find it very difficult to follow this rigid pattern of life that you set down for yourself, and that's really when you do get worried.

The regimentation of his life

> means getting up at a certain time and getting washed and dressed and that type of thing. You've got all the incidentals to think about, there's the clothing and the food and the shopping, and I don't like having to think, for instance, about what I'm going to have to eat because some days I find myself, my concentration is so bad that I can't even think of a satisfactory meal. And that's why I generally, I've got everything written down upstairs about food, what to buy in every week, because if I don't follow this pattern some weeks I'm not going to be able to get through that week without really great worry, and worry brings on stress, and stress brings on nervous debility and you don't know where you stand then, it's just a vicious ... and then you have to sort of rest up for three or four days until you gather enough mental energy back again. ... So you've got this for four days – I reckon it's

four days to a week – before you build up your mental strength again. And that's the reason I put everything down on paper because to survive a week ... it's almost as though your mind doesn't work properly, it's very dulled, very sluggish thinking and if it doesn't work. ... It's all a matter of survival, that's what it boils down to.

He sometimes feels that his mind needs a rest:

physically I'm not too bad, I can get about without much pain and effort, climbing stairs is no problem ... it's just mentally, you become exhausted mentally ... rather like an old person that requires one of those frames to get about, well occasionally I need a similar sort of frame to get about but it's not a physical frame, it's a mental frame, to enable me to get about.

Philip equivocates between the sense of worth that he receives from his present form of life and the strain that it imposes on him. Should he abandon this solitary project and seek admission to hospital or at the very least to a more sheltered form of accommodation, like a hostel? This is a question he frequently puts to himself but, on balance, he thinks not, for to do so would be to jettison the self-reliance on which he prides himself and also to jeopardise the social connections which he has so carefully fostered as an independent person. Presented with the option of an honourable retreat, Philip elects to soldier on.

Somewhat similar to Philip is Cyril. In his mid-fifties, Cyril first had a breakdown in his teens but subsequently married, and had a succession of jobs in mills, and then broke down again after his wife died eight years ago. He is now unemployed and cares for Sylvia, his mentally handicapped sister-in-law. His life is in obvious respects one of unmitigated hardship. Sylvia is severely retarded and cannot be left alone for more than half-an-hour. Cyril rarely leaves the house except to go to the shops – he describes himself as permanently 'on call' – and in the past year has been into the town centre only four times. He can hardly remember when he last left town. Every third week he spends £5.50 on a taxi to take him across town to the hospital; the taxi waits five minutes while he has his injection and then brings him home.

He receives a Night Attendance Allowance of £10 per week which it took him months to negotiate with the DHSS – he has a thick file of the correspondence – and he is now also trying to secure a Mobility Allowance. He can see another crisis on the horizon in that Sylvia's condition is deteriorating and even with assistance climbing the stairs gives her a good deal of pain, and he is now trying to negotiate a ground-floor flat with the Housing Department.

Cyril's life is entirely given over to Sylvia and her needs, but it is just in this that he has been able to recover a sense of value and purpose to his life. In a telling remark he says

> If anything, I would say that I've been trained for what I'm now doing in textiles. I was a supplier. Now Sylvia is my job. I'm *her* supplier. I meet her demands. Where in the weaving I might have had thirty weavers to see to, coming at me continuously, now it's gone down to one.
>
> Who meets *your* demands?
>
> I meet my own. There's only Norman the Samaritan that helps. I've got a social worker but she's not interested.

Cyril phones Norman once a week and after he had given him an account of what had happened to him over the past few months Norman told him (Cyril reported) that: 'What has happened to you since April is unbelievable. You must have a very strong will power to go through one crisis after another'.

As a result of the demands on him, Cyril finds himself in a constant cycle of debt. For example he experiences difficulty in paying for the television and has now taken out a loan with a finance company to pay for the licence; and he foresees that Sylvia will shortly need a new coat – she is a large size – for which he will need to increase his loan. Yet despite the pressures on his time, he also succeeds in generating a source of income – he has a knitting machine on which he knits hats and scarves and the previous week, for example, he had sold six sets of scarves and hats for £2 each. Just at the moment, however, his is unable to knit. The change in his medication which we described earlier, as well as making him drowsy, has produced a tremor which affects his writing and also the 'fiddly bits' in his knitting.

He feels bleak about the immediate future: 'I'm not happy at the moment, I'm in limbo'. In the longer term his hopes and aspirations – building a bungalow, for example – rest on the £2 to £3 which he spends each week on the pools, choosing teams on the basis of numbers which had held meaning for him in the past, for example 17–4–2–3 which was the number of a pattern when he was a weaver. The week before he won £5.23 and he has won small amounts on a number of previous occasions.

Caring for Sylvia in such a single-minded way is undoubtedly a lonely project and sometimes at night, after Sylvia has gone to bed,

Cyril sits on the steps and watches the couples walking by in the street and 'that's when it hurts'. He desires social contact and often leaves the doors of his house open so that neighbours can drop in and the previous week, for instance, a homeless woman had slept on his couch for a couple of nights. For Cyril himself most of the doors he needs to go through are closed, yet isolated and at the mercy of bureaucracies though he is, he values his life in caring for Sylvia:

I suppose I'd be at a loss without her.
How's that?
She keeps me going. [pause] There's always tomorrow!

In one sense Cyril's predicament is a case-study in social isolation, disability and poverty, yet seen in another way it is an example of the renewal and reconstruction of a life-project, of the rediscovery of purpose and value, in the face of the multiple devastations of mental breakdown, bereavement and job loss. It may also be helpful to view the relationship between Cyril and Sylvia in the light of the complaint from several of our participants that they always found themselves on the receiving end of relationships and lacked the opportunity to give.

Cosmology and value

Either in losing or in attempting to recover their sense of value, the majority of our participants measured their own fates by the standards of society at large. We can appreciate more readily the cultural roots of the evaluative frameworks in which most people interpreted their experience if we look at how a person strongly committed to the interpretation of personal and social life in the terms of a given cosmology experienced the sorts of personal and social displacements we have been describing. As it happens, one of the participants in this study whom we have not so far discussed was a young man who was an adherent of the Hare Krishna movement and we can see from his accounts that on all of the dimensions we have identified his experience is the reverse of that experienced by the secular majority.

Ray is quite different from any one else in our group in that he casts the problem of personhood in a spiritual dimension. Where what counts for the rest of our participants is membership of a human community, what counts for Ray is membership of a spiritual community. Where for everyone else the journey from ordinary living to mental-patienthood was a shocking displacement, for Ray it was a journey from a fallen state of personhood to a condition that promised access to

117

spiritual achievement. Ray recognises the category of 'mental illness' but feels at the same time that the experience of illness has brought him closer to the Lord. Where most people find themselves cut off, or even excommunicated, from social life through the experience of illness and its consequences, Ray has found himself brought into much closer relation with what he feels to be the true of community of believers. What for most people results in a form of exile has resulted for Ray in a form of discovery and communion.

From what he says, it is apparent that he recognises a vulnerability in himself – he speaks for example of his 'mental instability' – though as we shall describe his vulnerability has come to play an ennabling role in his spiritual journey. But it is plain that notions of burden and exclusion make no sense to him at all. Where for the secular majority the predicament of the ex-mental patient is experienced as a burden, and even as a source of shame, for Ray it is conceived as a form of virtue. Ray feels privileged to have had a schizophrenic breakdown and does not venture any of the complaints about exclusion or the depletion of social existence characteristic of the other participants. He lives in a room in an unstaffed hostel where he cooks for himself and manages quite happily on supplementary benefits: 'I'm not short of money. The Lord has provided me with everything really, a room, money, you name it!' Ray doesn't share any ordinary vices – he neither smokes nor drinks – nor does he experience his inability to afford the kinds of pleasures – to go to the cinema or to a disco for example – that are important to most people in his age group, as a loss.

Ray recognises different aspects of his behaviour as expressions of personal disturbance but at the same time sees them as contributing to a spiritual endeavour. Here, for example, is what he says about his attempt at suicide:

> Of course the Lord can wait for eternity for his souls to come back because he's not impatient. I was feeling impatient so I tried to commit suicide and get back to the Lord but he obviously didn't want me to go back quite so soon, so he saved my life and gave me these books to read. So I read them and hopefully I'll be cured and be able to, when I die, go back to the spiritual sky.
>
> What will you be cured of though, what do you want to be cured of?
>
> My rebelliousness against the Lord, that's the main reason I'm down here.
>
> Is that the same as your schizophrenia, though?

No, it's not.

Can you tell me the difference between your rebelliousness against the Lord and what we might call your schizophrenia? I'm asking a difficult question!

My schizophrenia is a symptom of mental instability but this mental instability can be a good thing in that because I'm mentally unstable I can worship the Lord so it must mean that the disease is really part of my religion. A very difficult question! . . . If I didn't have schizophrenia I'd be an ordinary person and I wouldn't have a relationship with the Lord, or try to come back to the Lord, and I'd carry out my life living a normal life, eating, sleeping, mating . . . that's what the animals do you see, and I believe that most people in this age, which is a degraded age, have forgotten all about the Lord and they just want to carry on enjoying themselves, enjoying their material senses.

Schizophrenia is perhaps, as Ray puts it, a 'form of the Lord's way of converting you back to worshipping him again'. Now that he is over the worst of his illness he claims to feel 'better' but it is apparent that in the context of his beliefs 'getting better' is an ambiguous achievement:

I think the better I feel the less contact I feel with the Lord. I think when I was very ill I was in much closer contact with the Lord than I am now, because now I feel better I feel more independent and I feel less dependent on the Lord, because when I was ill I was much more conscious that the Lord was there. The more ill I was, the more I was sure that there was a God but now I've got better the more my feeling that there is a God has weakened, so even though I'm physically much better, mentally much better from the point of view of coping with things, I'm not so in touch with the Lord any more.

For most people the experience of schizophrenia wreaks havoc in the continuity of their lives but not so for Ray:

I think it was part of my experience on earth which I was destined to have and the Lord must have decided it was a good thing for me to be mentally ill and to learn about him.

He enjoys the same sense of privilege in relation to his own future:

I see quite a bright light really. Because I'm mentally ill I don't have to go and work in one of those factories . . . or in one of those jobs where you have to work hard and gather learning from

119

working very hard and enjoying a sense of application. I can devote more time to the Lord than I would have done if I hadn't had schizophrenia.

Nor does he suffer the loneliness of exclusion common to many ex-mental patients:

> You could call it lonely but I've been alone for the past billion or so years, I've been by myself, so I don't feel that lonely and as it says 'You have the Lord in your heart', he lives in your heart. So I don't feel that lonely actually.

'WHAT YOU MEAN BY CONTENTMENT'

We have so far emphasised the continuity of the struggle that our participants faced but within it we can also identify points of repose or settlement. Jeffrey and Frank are examples of two older people – they are both over 50 – who after many years of upheaval have reached a point of settlement that for all the difficulties they still have to contend with they both find satisfactory. Much depends, as Jeffrey suggests, on 'what you mean by contentment'.

After six years or more in hostels, sheltered work-schemes and day centres Jeffrey's achievement as he defines it is to have cleared the psychiatric system. He feels lonely but he has reached the conclusion that loneliness is the price to be paid for having his own flat and living his own life to a much greater extent than heretofore on his own terms. In limited but vital ways he participates in a wider social life. He has a close friend whom he describes as a colleage – 'a colleague from the hospital' who 'goes to one of these day centres' – who comes to visit him regularly and often stays overnight. Recently they travelled down to Wembley together to see the Rugby League final and they are tentatively planning a trip to Paris in the autumn. Jeffrey has found out that the trip will cost £149 for four days which he thinks he could afford but he is worried that they won't have enough spending money left over to do the things they want to do when they are there, like going to a show. There are certain activities like swimming which he doesn't mind doing on his own, because 'swimming is more or less an individual sport isn't it?' but in the case of something like 'Wembley as a spectacle' he feels he can 'enjoy it more with someone going down' with him.

His other important relationship is with his elderly mother whom he visits most weekends, from Thursday or Friday through to Monday.

Jeffrey particularly values these visits because he feels he can be of some use:

> I'm kept quite occupied at my mother's . . . I do the lawns, I do the shopping for her, I get her breakfast ready, tea and supper, and she maybe gets the dinner ready.

He worries about what will happen when his mother dies, or if he loses the connection with his colleague, but for the time being these are the relationships that help sustain him. In the following Jeffrey conveys the double sense of a path that he has travelled and a point of settlement that has now been forced upon him and around which he can only circle:

> How do you see the future from where you've got to now?
> Well there's no future, it's a question of . . . .What have I done over the past ten years? Right, I know how the psychiatric system works, I know how these hostels work . . . I'm far better off than I was ten years ago.
> What do you mean when you say there's no future?
> Well, what future was there when I first went into hospital when I had no job? There's no future for me. You live from week to week, day to day. I mean, there's no prospect of a job for me . . . I mean, I'm turned 50 now. You're going round in a circle all the time, round and round.
> How could you get out of that circle? Or do you feel the circle is satisfactory, 'well that's the best for me at the moment' kind of thing?
> Well, it depends on what you mean by contentment doesn't it? . . . I mean if you're content to go and have a bet or an occasional drink or a meal in town – chicken and chips and peas and a pie – and going down to Wembley and going over to your mother's. . . . In a way that *is* contentment to me in my state of health. I mean, I have it better than most people have. I can consider myself luckier than a lot of people in these hostels who have suffered a mental breakdown of some description . . . I do, I consider myself lucky. I'm lonely, but this is partly with the fact that I've got my own flat now.

Frank has just turned 60 and since the age of 20 has spent about thirty years of his life either in mental hospitals or in prison. He realises in retrospect that his illness started when he was in the army at the end of the Second World War and he saw a vision which he tried to attack with a bayonet. After the war he married and attempted to start a job, but 'odd feelings' and voices would come upon him as he set off for work and he would wander off, sometimes for weeks at a time, living rough and in spikes. After two years he saw a psychiatrist and was admitted to hospital on a voluntary basis. He was treated with unmodified ECT, insulin coma and drugs; after three months he was discharged with, by his own account, his symptoms much increased. His delusions and hallucinations made it impossible for him to work, and the financial problems which resulted led to constant arguments with his wife. Over a fifteen-year period he received a number of prison sentences for violent assault, including a spell of eight years in Dartmoor after he had attacked a woman and nearly killed her.

After he last came out of hospital seven years ago Frank was dispatched to a large inner-city hostel for homeless people, one of those places, as he described, into which 'the dregs and the sweepings' are put, 'to keep them out of the way'. Frank couldn't stand the place, it was

absolute chaos in there – the police coming in in the early hours of the morning and dragging people out. I'd have done something really bad if I'd stayed there!

Eventually a worker from a voluntary agency helped him find a flat on the ground floor of a block of flats for single people, all in their late fifties and sixties, on a small estate. 'I was', he said, 'so glad when I got this flat'. Yet pleased though he was, Frank did not have much more to his name than the clothes he stood up in and he found himself forced to live in his new flat for ten weeks without furniture – from November through to January – before a social worker visited him. Frank now has one or two pieces of furniture but he still cannot afford a television or a fridge. He draws his benefit on a Monday and finds that by Saturday he is down to coppers, and over the weekends lives on bread and dripping. The flat is quiet, which Frank likes, but there is a large council estate down the road and local youths have twice broken Frank's windows after the pubs have closed and on weekends he now sits up on guard till the early hours of the morning.

He often speaks of the 'loneliness of survival' and sometimes thinks that he might be better off in 'a nice hostel'. He has been hearing 'funny voices' since he was about 10 and they still pester him periodically. Sometimes, for example, he finds himself talking or shouting to the voice when he is on a bus. He also says that he does a lot of shouting when he is in the flat on his own and he knows that people roundabout think of him as a 'queer bugger' and fight shy of him – 'they put you out on a limb'.

Yet despite his poverty and isolation, and the upheavals of his history, Frank manages, quite surprisingly perhaps, to convey a sense of dignity and value, as a person who has withstood and come through. He has, as he describes, lived 'a very violent life' but he has now learned to 'channel that thing'. Sometimes, he says, 'you get an inward tension in your mind' and he knows that 'there's a hate there'. Not so long ago when the tension came upon him he would have hit somebody but now when he starts to feel angry he takes a long walk in the country – sixteen miles or more – to tire himself out. And one of the pleasures of walking in the country, as he describes, is that unlike his neighbours in the town strangers will stop and talk to him.

Frank doesn't have any close friends, but to help relieve his loneliness he has what he calls 'a secret', a 'nice lady' whom he visits once a month for £10. He has attended local meetings of the National Schizophrenia Fellowship but found the group 'stagnant': 'The "sufferers", as they call them, don't get much out of it'. He sometimes goes to a MIND centre, which he quite enjoys, but feels a bit patronised by middle-class ladies there 'doing good', like the magistrate's wife who makes the tea. The activity he enjoys most (though he sometimes has to go short of food to support it) is to buy a 'Weekly Rover' pass for about £5.50 and to spend sometimes the whole day travelling on buses and local trains. For Frank this is the most feasible way he knows to combat isolation – he chats to people he meets on the buses and trains – and to feel that he is in some sense part of the life of the wider society. It is, in a limited but still direct and genuine sense, a way of being in society as an alternative to marginalisation.

Rather like Jeffrey, Frank feels that he is better off than a lot of people and that he enjoys a certain kind of happiness. He has come to accept himself in the strong sense of learning to *like* himself the way he is:

I know I'll never be a normal person, but I don't want to. I wouldn't know what to do. I'd be alienated from what I've become through being like this so long. What I am now is my normality.

He knows his own limitations and strengths:

I don't ask for much now. I just want to get through – no big upheavals! I just want to manage in life in the years I've got left. I've been through so much that nothing can touch me now.

6

BEN: ONE PERSON'S JOURNEY

In this chapter we offer an extended example of one person's journeying that throws into sharp relief many of the issues we have discussed: the continuity of the struggle; the combination of reversals and advances; the reflections and revaluations that these provoke; the work that has to be done to repair the damage of a set-back; the dilemmas that present themselves at each point along the way; and perhaps most importantly the whole problem for the ex-mental patient in re-establishing his credibility as a person.

In an important sense this is a hopeful story of a journey from displacement and rootlessness to social participation and membership. And so in a way it is – the story of one man's courage and tenacity. But through Ben's description of his vicissitudes we can glimpse the complex of social and cultural forces that impinge upon the life of the ex-mental patient. Ben recognises that there is that about him which puts him in jeopardy when under stress. The central problem in his trial is to find ways of managing his stress, and have it acknowledged by other people, without finding that his credibility as a person is put in question. In Ben's experience, knowledge of his psychiatric past means that when he displays signs of stress he is at once vulnerable to speedy redefinition as a mental patient. What Ben wants from others is a more robust view of his strengths and capabilities as a person in which his vulnerabilities are acknowledged by others in the context of support for his enterprise – for what he is trying to achieve. As Ben feels, in virtue of his psychiatric history all too often people react precipitately and inappropriately, overlook his strengths, and under-estimate his capacities to help himself. And he then has once more to renew the struggle to re-establish his credibility.

Ben does not come from Northtown and before he arrived there had lived a rootless existence for some years, interspersed with a number of admissions to hospital. He fetched up in the town on his wanderings largely by chance, was admitted to hospital under section and, after his discharge, decided to stay in the town and try and make something of his life there. He describes how he made a conscious decision to attempt to lift himself out of the condition of isolation and acute personal misery in which, for a long time, he had felt himself locked:

> I made myself become integrated into society, if you like, into *groups*, I suppose I consciously did this because I'd become completely isolated and I was just wandering the countryside really, I was just down-and-out.

Many years before he had worked for a charity and he decided while he was in hospital that

> I would remake that part of my life because I'd cut myself off from that kind of activity.

For Ben, remaking this part of his life meant putting himself in contact with various local groups. Over time he got to know a number of people there:

> They had friends, and they had neighbours and things, and they invited me to baby-sit and then they invited me to tea . . . and then we just became friends, and I got to know their friends, and from there I've moved out to do other things. That's how it's kind of spread, and so I've got to know people. . . . But I felt I *had* to do that . . . because being unemployed you can just about meet nobody and have no friends, especially in the position I was in.

Working himself out of his isolated position has not been easy. As we described earlier, after he was discharged from hospital he spent a year in a hostel and was then allocated a council flat on a large housing estate. For the first three years that he lived there

> I didn't get to know any of my neighbours, nobody round there at all. I didn't feel at all integrated into the estate, I felt very lonely and very frightened in lots of ways.

Then a year ago

> a video shop became vacant, just about the time of the elections, and I decided to . . . I got a petition together to use it as a community shop and community centre, and since then we have

125

formed a community association and I've got to know me neighbours. It's an excuse – it could have been anything else, it just happened to be a very handy thing and I got to know the people upstairs and the people who own the flat next door and the people down the road. . . . We've got agreement from the Housing Department for us to have it on a nominal rent but we need some more money before we can open it.

Ben has been remarkably successful:

At the last meeting there was about twenty people there and a councillor I went to talk to said, 'if you get twelve people to a meeting you'll be doing well', and I think I'm doing quite well really with twenty people from the estate. Representatives from the housing offices and social services have turned up, and they've given us a small grant. So we've got support for the idea. The social workers I've talked to, and the housing department, both think it's a good idea. They've been waiting, really, for it to happen in the community, so I just happened to be in the right spot.

At the same time he has misgivings about being the initiator of such an ambitious venture:

In some ways I think I would have much preferred to have joined one because it is bloomin hard work and worry trying to create a social entity, especially as people don't really want to talk about constitutions and things – I can't really say that *I* want to spend a lot of my time delving into things like that but. . . . People come back and say, 'When's the shop opening?', people come to me and say that, and I say 'Well, we've still got some things to do yet'.

There are two distinct parts to Ben's life, and hence two distinct ways of describing him. One is to describe him as someone who has been part of, and as we shall see is still part of, what ex-mental patients call the 'psychiatric system'. The other is to describe him as a form of community activist. Ben sees these areas of his life as largely separate from one another but at points they overlap and it is apparent from what he says that he has been able to turn his membership in the one to good social and political account in the other:

they *do* overlap. One person on the community association is an ex-mental patient himself whom I got to know in hospital and he himself is a community kind of activist, if you like, and he works at a community centre as an outreach worker and so he's been very valuable in suggesting ideas and getting ideas for grants and things. So they do overlap and I've also recruited patients to give out leaflets for the Labour Party and things like that.

Ben has, then, in a number of decisive moves, pushed himself out from the lonely and isolated predicament of the ex-mental patient into the thick of social action. In important measure, he has succeeded in re-establishing his credibility and in reconstituting himself as a person who is not primarily defined by his psychiatric history. Yet, as he has now discovered, to recover lost ground is one thing, to hold on to it quite another. As Ben describes, his very success in lifting himself out of his isolation has caused 'another problem, one from being isolated to one of pressure'. The project he has generated is a constant worry:

I worry a lot about it. There's this form sat on my desk for a month really and eventually I knew it had to be in for the grant ... and I worried because I needed some help to get a good application and I couldn't get proper accounts together, and somehow it never got together. In the end I just sat down and said, 'I've just go to do this, no matter what. It's got to get in!' So I sat down and did it and got it in in a rush. It's not the best application in the world, really, but I'm hoping that at least I've got it in on time and that they might come back and say, 'Well, you've got to firm up your ideas a bit'. So sometimes I do sit and worry instead of doing something. . . . It's not easy to work in the community, to work on an estate ... I've recruited just who I could but they don't really get on together. One comes to me and says 'That bloomin so-and-so!'

Having advanced so far, last year Ben experienced a reversal and was readmitted to hospital under section. Until then he thought that he had broken free of the psychiatric system:

I thought I'd got rid of it. I'd been out of hospital for four years now, I was going along fine and there'd been no problems. This last year it really upset me going back into hospital. . . . Up till last year I thought really that the hospital had cured me if you like, I was cured.

Ben was himself aware that he had been labouring under the pressure of his new station and had come to his own decision that he wanted to consult a doctor. In particular he was having a problem sleeping which had made him a 'bit edgy', as he put it:

> The sleep problem comes from the worry and the work that I'm doing and the things that I'm involved in, the exhaustion if you like, and the ideas that I have and not getting things done – all these worries come together. In other words it's not just in my chemistry, it's to do with the life that I lead.

While Ben recognised his own stress he felt, nevertheless, that he could be helped to manage it in his own person and that he did not merit redefinition as a mental patient. However, friends who were acquainted with his history thought otherwise and took him into hospital.

> I feel they overreacted because I had sleeping tablets in my pocket and I needed sleep as much as anything. The thing is, when I take those tablets I might sleep late, but it does give me a good night's rest and stops me from getting into really bad problems. It's becoming a common occurrence now, the sleep problem and the subsequent going into hospital – for the last three times it has been that cause.

Ben would have preferred an alternative course of action:

> I think, to accept my solution of taking some tablets and having a sleep would be a lot better, and they would realise that if it didn't work after a good night's sleep, and I was still poorly, *then* they could take me in.

He describes how the person with a history of mental illness easily becomes vulnerable to redefinition as a mental patient:

> You see, the problem is you can just look at me now, you can go next door, ring up, and you could have me in hospital on your word, not on my word. That is the problem and I could say 'I protest, I protest, I'm all right!' And I *would* protest, because I am all right. And you could say 'No he isn't!', and you might have your own reasons for doing that. That's the problem of hospitalisation and you would be doing it in the best of hearts – I'm not suggesting it's not concern. . . . But I don't always like being in hospital . . . and if there is some credence to helping people in the community, it's no good when there's a problem just sending people into hospital. There has to be a solution other than that, I think.

Ben evinces the difficulty which many ex-mental patients experience in securing a hearing for themselves as agents who are knowledgeable about their own conditions. Ben's achievements in reconstituting himself as a credible person are considerable but his innate vulnerabilities coupled with the knowledge which others possess of his psychiatric history render him easily liable to redefinition as someone incapable of making rational decisions about his own well-being. While he would have preferred to negotiate an understanding as to how he could be helped to manage his stress in his own person, at the same time he recognises the awkward problems of judgement that are involved:

It's a bit like being drunk, being mentally ill, because a drunken driver will say 'Oh, I'm quite all right, I can drive!', and it's as difficult, probably, talking to me when I have basically not had any sleep. . . . And so when people talk to me then, it's like talking to a drunken man in some ways and they have to make a decision on my behalf and they do do it in all good intentions but because people are deferential they defer to the doctor, and the doctor says, 'Oh he's mentally ill, he's got this. Give him this injection and then everything will be all right'.

Ben did not dispute that he was incapacitated and in need of rest, and that, to a degree, he needed others to take charge of him. What he did dispute was the display of power whereby he precipitately found himself organised back into the mental patient frame. The pressure of the situation – Ben's difficulties in communicating when under stress and the fears of those around him – made the renegotiation of understanding that he would have preferred impossible for him to carry through. He therefore gave in to the pressure on him to succumb to a redefinition of what he felt to be a manageable disturbance:

The last time I was in the hospital I said 'I surrender' . . . To do with the mental illness I surrender, because I just can't get any sense out of it. I mean, if people come along and say 'Oh Ben you've got to go into hospital', I just say 'All right, I'll go in' and if they jab me with drugs and send me to hell which they *have* done, I just have to pray that I get out of it.

When he finds himself redefined as a mental patient:

I don't know what to do. I don't know whether to fight or to sit quietly and let it happen. And sometimes I fight and sometimes I flight. It's difficult to know what to do. Because if you fight in the

129

hospital they'll give you an injection and you're out and can't do a thing. . . . It's an incredibly difficult problem in the hospital to know what to do.

Ben may have been uncertain whether to 'fight or flight' in the hospital but in the event he engaged in a bit of both to good effect. After he was sectioned, he was for the first time shown his rights as a patient:

> I'd never seen them before, so I kept them, and it said I could write to the hospital managers or the tribunal in Nottingham. So I wrote . . . I wrote saying I wanted to be taken off the section as quickly as possible to get back to work, and that I would co-operate in any way possible. They did take me off section, and I did go back to work when they suggested.

Ben's abrupt reversal had considerable effects on the relationships he had established:

> It was upsetting with the friends I had made in the town independent of the hospital. Some of them knew that I had been in hospital, a lot of them didn't. For me to go into hospital and have them visit me, that was upsetting. I felt, if you like, I'd grown in self-confidence in certain things and it was a reduction, it was a step backwards. . . . I like people to feel 'Oh, he's all right' but I now have to convince them that I'm all right because of that. For me to have this relapse or whatever it was, I then had to re-establish that I'm kind of all right.

For example

> With friends, when I went in again, it has taken quite a long time to build up trust. Just little things, like baby-sitting, and it was five or six months before they would ask me again. Because they were worried – there was just this bit of 'We had better not'.

The most important aspect of the repair work that he found he had to do in his relationships was 'building up that trust, that feeling again'. It all comes back, as Ben puts it, to the problem of stigma, of getting over the barrier of people 'thinking that you're mad because you've been in a mental hospital':

> Trying to get over that – that I'm all right, I'm a functioning being, that I can actually take part in a committee or be a chairman of a committee, that I can get some money in and I won't go and spend it somewhere! It's building up that kind of

trust. It's a trust that you have to build up with any kind of human being anyway, but I feel that I've got that extra obstacle.

He has been able to recover a good deal of ground:

As people get to know me, they make contact and come to expect things from me and I expect things from them. They know the kinds of things I can do. Usually, and certainly in the kindest possible way, people know I have had an illness and say 'Don't let yourself get too pressured!' and although they are reacting to me in my illness, I certainly don't think they are doing it in any kind of malevolent way, they are doing it in a 'We know if you do too much, or get too pressured, then you are going to have a problem' kind of way, and they are very kind about that, people who know.

In Ben's case people are able to 'react to him in his illness' as he nicely puts it, and still treat and respect him as an ordinary and capable human being. That he should be able to say this is a measure of his own achievement for there are, as we have seen, formidable cultural obstacles to this kind of integration. For most people who have had a schizophrenic illness, to be 'reacted to in their illness' is to find themselves swiftly reincorporated into an alien set of categories.

Nevertheless he still has suspicions to contend with. Recently, for example, he has been given a job on a Community Programme. Over the past week he has been feeling a bit depressed and his employer has told him to take time off work. According to Ben, his employer's worry is that his depression is connected to his illness and that he has returned to work too quickly after his discharge from hospital:

When I went for an interview, and filled in the form, I didn't put on it that I'd had a mental illness because I'd tried two interviews before and I believed that I just wouldn't get even an interview if I put mental illness on it, so I didn't. I was employed, and he was quite happy with me, and I think he's still happy with me, but when I came back after the recent illness he said that he thought I wasn't ready and gave me time off with pay until he could have a word with the doctor about it. So I'm not on the sick but I've got time off.

As far as Ben is concerned, his depression is a form of ordinary despondency brought about by the trials he has had to go through in re-establishing his credibility after he came out of hospital. He appreciates his employer's concerns but feels that the nature and scale of the burden he has to contend with in trying to make his way in social life is insufficiently understood. In Ben's experience the ex-mental patient is tainted by his history of illness such that what for most people would pass as workaday depression or eccentricity is often perceived as a sign of illness. It is perhaps this aspect of his wider experience that he finds to be the most intractable:

> That's the worrying aspect of it, the stigma . . . and I really don't know how to cope with that, I really don't know how to cope.

A problem has also occurred over his driving licence since he came out of hospital:

> My licence comes up every three years – because I've had this mental illness – for renewal and they've refused it, so I can't use the car any more. And that's added pressure, because when I've got a car I can use it – if I'm a bit late I can get in there. But they've stopped my licence and I can't have a car for six months. I'm intending to appeal on this, because I'm a very good driver, I've never had an accident.

Ben is angry at having to deal with this new problem alongside everything else:

> I'm just fed up with the stigma attached to the illness.
> That's a manifestation of it?
> Yes, it must be. I'm absolutely fed up with it because I'm a good driver and I know that when I'm ill I don't drive the car.
> How do you make that sort of decision?
> I take advice from the people around me.
> So, if someone says to you, 'Should you really be driving?'
> Yes, if someone gives me that signal, then I'll take it.

Ben describes himself as a Christian and feels that it is, perhaps, his faith which helps to keep him going. He has a definite sense of mission:

> I'd like to be a Lenin or something! In some kind of way, I'd like to be a socialist reformer and do something really significant but as I've grown older I've come to realise that that really isn't to be . . . I don't think I'll ever really achieve anything of any great importance but I just kind of concentrate on small things.

His experience over the past year has changed the way in which he thinks about himself:

Feeling now the way I do today, I don't feel it would happen again, but I felt that for the last four years, and just last year I went in again . . . and it's happened periodically since 1971. And so this last time I went in, I've really kind of come to terms with myself – that it could happen again, and I keep on guard. . . . I do see myself as a person that's had a mental problem and could quite well have it again.

He intends to keep going in what he has set out to do but he is under no illusions about the future:

I don't know, I can see it as being as hard as ever, probably get harder as the pressures build up.

7

THE PERSON (MENTAL PATIENT) PREDICAMENT

What, then, do we learn from our participants about the social fate of the person with a history of schizophrenic illness? We shall start by summarising what seems to us some of the key issues that have emerged and then proceed to some suggestions for the kinds of conceptual frameworks we need to engage with the concerns of ex-mental patients. Finally we shall attempt to locate our discussion within the wider bearings of contemporary mental health policy and provide a tentative sketch of the predicament of the person with a history of mental illness in social life.

DISCONNECTION

Most of our participants were able to forge some form of connection or life-line that kept them going and helped maintain some at least minimal sense of the integrity of their life projects. Though they lived alone many of our participants were in contact with at least one relative who proved important in a variety of ways, both material and emotional. Some people derived a source of satisfaction from looking after pets: Bill has his dog, William his parrot and cats, and Barry a budgie and pet mice. Having responsibility for pets, Barry said, helped keep him from suicide. Sometimes to their surprise, after a succession of bad experiences with Joe Public, participants were able to develop a supportive connection with a sympathetic neighbour. So, for example, Barry had got to know the neighbours across the road and used to go over every morning for half-an-hour for a chat, and he was even invited to spend Christmas Day with them. Ian described how the couple next door had been very good to him and sold him a suite for next to nothing and helped him out in numerous small ways.

But to a considerable extent these were moments of relief within a wider experience of disconnection and structural isolation. In the structural spheres of housing and employment in particular participants generally found themselves powerless to influence their fates and felt they had no choice but to accept (and be grateful) for what was given them. Jeffrey felt he had to 'comply with the rules – "Right, you have to go into a hostel!"'. Bill, Henry and Frank, for example, were placed in vandal-prone ground-floor flats where Bill waited four years for his electricity to be connected, and Frank ten weeks through the bleak winter months before a social worker visited him to arrange a grant for furniture. The poverty of lives led on welfare benefits enforced a competition over basic necessities that could prove detrimental to people's health. Often enough a visit to the cinema, or a night out with friends, would mean a sandwich for dinner. Budgets were maintained under a tight rein, everything worked out to the last penny, with little scope for contingency, a new pair of boots or a coat for the winter. With social security, as Ben put it, 'you can just about manage to trundle along'.

Friendships, as we have seen, were as vital as they were tenuous. Time and again participants reported a vicious circle in which lack of resources coupled with the burden of their psychiatric histories exacerbated such difficulties as they already had in making and sustaining friendships. A further effect of their structural isolation was on mobility. Ben and Henry had their cars and Frank his 'Weekly Rover' pass in which he invested a considerable proportion of his scant resources, but participants repeatedly complained how difficult it was for them to find the wherewithal to escape from the sites of their daily lives. 'I'd love to see the ocean again', said Barry, 'even if it's only for a day'. For those who did manage to escape, a holiday was always a tremendous boost in the trials that faced them. Thus Ian had organised with two friends, also ex-mental patients, to rent a caravan by the seaside for a week and felt, he said, 'very anti-depressed' when he got back; he plans to go again next year.

A special difficulty for our participants was to surmount an identity as a mental patient. Even where participants might be said to have 'got better' their credibility was easily put in question. At best they had a precarious foothold in ordinary life in which their personhood was constantly on probation and they were required to provide repeated demonstrations that they were normal and there was nothing untoward about them. And a relapse invariably meant that another round of repair work had to be underaken. Though they were several of them active strategists in their own care, and could in an important sense be said to be their own main carers, their potential as human beings capable of giving as much as receiving was generally disregarded. Philip identified a shared desire to make a mark, to achieve some form of recognition, when he spoke of the importance of being able to 'make a difference to something, affect something'.

Ben described how some people were able to 'react to him in his illness' and still treat and respect him as a person of worth who was not primarily defined by his illness. But this was very much the limiting case, and 'reacting to people in their illness' generally meant viewing them in their difference as denizens of an alien sphere of being. Disclosure of a psychiatric history incurred the risk of being made to feel 'less of a person'. Typical was Henry's experience at the Job Centre where he found staff to be 'nervy because they know you're schizophrenic, as though they feel. "What's he going to do next?"'. It would appear, indeed, that the term 'schizophrenia' is often freighted with such denigratory meaning that the perception of the person is distorted, in Henry's apt phrase, 'completely out of perspective', and people are brought to think 'all sorts from different corners'.

It is apparent that the pressure to conceal their psychiatric histories also contributed to participants' stress. Though they eschewed identification as mental patients, at the same time most of them sought recognition and acceptance of their vulnerabilities as facets of the sorts of people they had turned out to be. In addition concealment brought with it the problem of how to account for yawning gaps in the narratives of their lives.

Participants appeared to have received little or no guidance in tackling the meanings of schizophrenia and negotiating the cultural burden which the diagnosis inflicted on them. They had as best they could to become their own guides and try to put 'bits together to realise what it means'. The social world often appeared strange and threatening, assumptions and expectations that could previously have been taken for granted were unsettled, and participants found themselves trying to find orientation, and groping for answers as to what makes life worth living, in a seemingly inauspicious set of structural conditions. In crucial respects they were in the position of travellers in a strange country, equipped with only a very rudimentary map for guidance, trying to make their way through a web of uncertainty and ambiguity in which each path concealed a snare and frequently led nowhere in particular.

Though the terms of life offered by psychiatric day care were often judged a dead-end, just one day following the next, without sense or purpose, going it alone was recognised to be a high-risk enterprise.

Above all, participants wanted access to opportunities that promised to lead somewhere and enable them to establish a direction to their lives. Most of them would not have gone along with Terence's remark that the schizophrenic should be left alone to see visions and hear voices as he pleases, not because they necessarily disagreed with the ethic he espoused but simply because their urges did not take them that way – they did not *want* to pass their lives sitting in a room seeing visions and listening to voices.

DIFFERENCE OR MEMBERSHIP?

If we try to single out two distinct points of emphasis in what our participants tell us, one is perhaps given in Ben's remark about the difficulty of 'getting over the barrier of people thinking you're mad because you've been in a mental hospital'; and another in Henry's assertion that 'with schizophrenia you're not living, you're just existing . . . I think schizophrenia will always make me a second-class citizen'.

The first of these has to do with how ex-mental patients are commonly perceived by society at large, the tendency for them to be identified largely in the vocabulary of difference rather than of membership; the second with material constraints on participation in social life, the tendency for ex-mental patients to be marginalised or even pauperised. Taken together they locate the social fate of the ex-mental patient within the twin themes of identity and structure and bring into sharp focus two distinct but closely interconnected ways of being shut out from membership of the larger society, two facets of a process of devaluation that is exhibited not only in how people are seen or represented but also in the structural options made available to them.

From what our participants tell us it would appear that the experience of devaluation is one of the key issues that concerns them. What, perhaps, they can be said to ask of us is that we should relocate the discussion of the lives of people with a history of mental illness in the community away from 'illness' (the management of an illness and the management of patients) as the dominant frame of reference to the frame of 'well-being', which puts personhood rather than patienthood in the foreground of analysis. As we have seen our participants wanted to help in resisting becoming entrapped in a condition of mental patienthood, a form of exclusion in which people with a history of mental illness are established largely in their difference and exiled to the margins of social life.

137

As the conventional designation of them as 'the mentally ill' brings out, we have tended to see people with mental illness as secondary sorts of people and to discuss the issues in terms of competing ways of dealing with such secondary people. The questions that specially concern our participants, therefore, are not so much medical questions as questions relating to a broader understanding of their well-being and their place in a moral community. It was not so much that medical perspectives were seen to be unimportant as that these were just part of such a wider understanding and taken by themselves could not adequately tackle the problems of ex-mental patients in social life. Considered as mental patients, people with mental illness may receive exemplary treatment but clearly such treatment will of itself do little to address the complex questions of valuation that concern them.[1]

PERSON–DISORDER INTERACTIONS

It may help to clarify the argument for a frame of reference that is not bound by questions of illness or disorder if we turn briefly to some recent studies of person–disorder interactions among people with a history of schizophrenic illness which introduce a conceptual distinction between the person and the disorder. John Strauss, Professor of Psychiatry at Yale University, describes how the interest in such interactions arises 'from one major lesson that people with severe mental illness appear to be trying to teach us'. This lesson

> is reflected in a question once posed by one of our subjects. During an interview early in our research, she said, 'Why don't you ever ask what I do to help myself?' What she and others suggest is that the person as an active agent interacts with mental disorder in a crucial way that influences the course of the disorder. Thus, in contrast to some models of mental illness ... my hypothesis is that the role of the person in mental disorder is not peripheral, merely as a passive victim of a disease to be fixed by medicine.[2]

In a series of interviews with people who had improved after ten years or more of serious mental disorder, several participants described a change in attitude that in retrospect was a key turning-point in their illness careers:

> Somehow, after an extended period, they found themselves

wanting not just to live with their illness but to have a life along with it or in spite of it. Some stated that they came to accept their disorders. But this was not the kind of giving-up acceptance or resignation that often seems generated by the attempts some professionals make at helpful teaching (e.g. 'You have an illness like diabetes and will have it all your life. You'll need to stay on medication and there are certain things you'll never be able to do'). The acceptance described by these subjects was one that involved hope for a better life and the resolve to work for it.[3]

In a complementary study Sue Estroff found that most of her subjects were willing to acknowledge signs of illness, yet at the same time what

they resist and reject are notions that those signs mean they are incompetent, failed or somehow revised individuals because of these problems. Many make what we call 'normalising statements' in order, we hypothesise, to stress and reassert their similarities with others and to retain claim to their persisting, unrecognised, not-disordered selves.[4]

The position of many of her subjects, Estroff suggests, is captured by the re-mark of an ex-mental patient: 'You are not your illness! Find another role besides mental patient!'[5] She is brought to the ironic conclusion that

the loss and disorder of person so characteristic of our conceptions of schizophrenia may be at least partly our own invention, and one of the many ways in which we desert the person who has schizophrenia. . . . *Becoming a schizophrenic* is essentially a social and interpersonal process, not an inevitable consequence of primary symptoms and neurochemical abnormality.[6]

PERSONHOOD AND ORDINARY LIFE

But what is involved in bringing the concepts of the person and of personhood into the foreground of analysis? In order to do justice to the experience of our participants, what we need is a framework which can tackle the experience of exile we have described both in its structural and moral dimension. Some help in this direction is to be found in a recent discussion by the philosopher, Charles Taylor, of the moral enterprise of human lives in which he locates the understanding of personhood within the struggle of agents to be 'rightly placed' in relation to the good. Human lives, Taylor suggests, are led in a space of moral concerns that involves not so much moral issues in a narrow sense as crucial discriminations around what makes life worth living. In our own period the notion of 'ordinary life' has come to take on a particular significance:

> The notion that there is a certain dignity and worth in this life requires a contrast; no longer, indeed, between this life and some 'higher' activity like contemplation, war, active citizenship or heroic asceticism, but now lying between different ways of living the life of production and reproduction. The notion is never that *whatever* we do is acceptable. That would be unintelligible as the basis for a notion of human dignity. Rather the key point is that the higher is to be found not outside of but as a *manner of living* ordinary life.[7]

On Taylor's account we can understand the enterprise of human lives only in respect of people's efforts at orientation within the space of such strong discriminations or what he also terms the space of questions about the good. From this point of view, then, selfhood and the good are inextricably intertwined themes. As Taylor puts it, 'we are only selves insofar as we move in a certain space of questions, as we seek and find an orientation to the good'.[8] To invoke the metaphor of orientation in space is to think of selves as constituted in a moral space within which they have to try to find their way and we thus need to understand our predicament in terms of finding or losing orientation in such a space. Being a self 'is inseparable from existing in a space of moral issues, to do with identity and how one ought to be. It is being able to find one's standpoint in this space, being able to occupy, to *be* a perspective in it.'[9] There is an essential link between identity and orientation in moral space:

> To know who you are is to be oriented in moral space, a space in which questions arise about what is good or bad, what is worth doing and what not, what has meaning and importance for you and what is trivial and secondary.[10]

In Taylor's account, the question of orientation in relation to the good is 'essential to being a functional human agent' and represents a 'craving which is ineradicable from human life'.[11] Issues about the worth, or weight, or substance of our lives are thus implicated in the question of 'how I am "placed" or "situated" in relation to the good, or whether I am in "contact" with it',[12] and this question is of 'crucial and inescapable concern for us', for 'we cannot but strive to give our lives meaning or substance'.[13] Furthermore the issue of 'our condition can never be exhausted for us by what we *are*, because we are always also changing and *becoming*.'[14] The question that concerns us is not only where we *are*, but also where we're *going*:

> Since we cannot do without an orientation to the good, and since we cannot be indifferent to our place relative to this good, and since this place is something that must always change and become, the issue of the direction of our lives must arise for us.[15]

Similarly the question of the sense of the good, and where a person is placed in relation to it, must be woven into the person's understanding of his or her life as an unfolding story, as a 'quest'. Making sense of our lives as a story is also, like orientation to the good, an essential feature of human lives. Because 'we cannot but orient ourselves to the good, and thus determine our place relative to it and hence determine the direction of our lives, we must inescapably understand our lives in narrative form, as a "quest".'[16]

From this sketch of Taylor's argument we can perhaps be helped to clarify both what our participants are up to in their various 'doings' and 'beings', and to identify more firmly some of the obstacles and constraints they are battling against. In the first place we are now able to locate the strivings of people with a history of mental illness within a more developed understanding of the moral enterprise of human lives. We can begin to see that what our participants are engaged in is a version of an enterprise that is not peculiar to ex-mental patients but is common to all human lives, and that the concepts in which we endeavour to describe and understand them must therefore be precisely those that we use to try to give an adequate account of other people's 'doings' and 'beings'.

Second, Taylor helps us to clarify the special difficulties that ex-mental patients experience in what we have described as the effort to re-establish their personhood. The concept of the person, it has been argued, properly identifies not just a natural kind like 'human being' as much as beings whose existence has a particular value and importance. Persons 'are beings with the capacity to value their own existence'.[17] The concept of personhood embraces this understanding of the person but possesses additional force and points us towards what is involved in being a person and realising the capacity to value one's own existence. In Charles Taylor's terms, it invites us to look at the options and constraints which different groups of people confront in attempting to satisfy their craving to be 'rightly placed' in relation to the good.

From the standpoint of our participants we can define the good in broad terms as the opportunity to participate, in Taylor's phrase, in a manner of ordinary living that they judged worthwhile and that lent point to their lives. With the exception of Ray who identified the enterprise of his life as a spiritual quest, this is the emphasis that our participants gave to the quest of their lives. Opportunity here involves in equal measure questions of identity and material questions. To give an account of what it means to move (or not) within the space of the good is necessarily also to give an account of what, in the terms of a given set of valuations, it means to move (in the strong sense of belong or participate) in the space of social life.

In crucial respects the accounts of our participants evince an ambiguity or uncertainty about where they are now placed in relation to the good and often a definite sense of exile or separation from it. It is, of course, evident that the deprivations which participants described implicated a variety of goods and no one in particular may be accorded special significance, but taken together they make up that bundle that we call participation in ordinary life. Participants drew upon a cluster of terms to describe the experience of exile or separation from the good but perhaps predominant among them was the sense that the worth of their lives had been put in question and that they were perceived by others (and sometimes brought to judge themselves) as useless.

The testimonies we have examined abound in details of the material and existential difficulties in orientation in the space of the good that were borne upon participants by the barriers that were put in the way of their particpation in social life. Formally, the person with a history of mental illness does not cease to be a person but it would appear that he or she often becomes a very marginal and questionable person. It is evident that the realisation of personhood – of equality of regard and entitlement, feeling that one exists as a person of value and is not *primarily* defined as a mental patient – is a very precarious and fragile achievement that often involves prolonged struggle. Shifting the frame of reference from mental patienthood to personhood helps us to bring the question of where people with a history of mental illness are placed in relation to the good into sharp relief and to understand a little more clearly the nature of the quest in which they are involved.

THE PERSON (MENTAL PATIENT) PREDICAMENT

Exile from the good is readily enough understood in the context of what Ralf Dahrendorf has recently termed the modern social conflict in which the claims of wealth creation outweigh those of citizenship and entitlements for the many give place to provisions for the few. The emphasis on growth and enterprise has generated a social category of people (sometimes referred to as the underclass) who find themselves in persistent poverty and are 'separated from the rest by what amount to entitlement barriers'.[18] The modern social conflict is about 'attacking inequalities which restrict full civic participation by social, economic or political means, and establishing the entitlements which make up a rich and full status of citizenship'.[19]

Broadly we can locate the vicissitudes of people with mental illness within the antagonisms Dahrendorf describes but there is an additional twist we need to consider which derives from the direction of contemporary mental health policies. The experiences of our Northtown participants may, perhaps, point to some important features in the wider predicaments of people with mental illness in societies presently undergoing the transition from hospital to community based forms of care. In the American context Dan Lewis and his colleagues have recently provided an ironic and incisive account of the 'prolonged and turbulent transformation of the mental system' brought about by deinstitutionalisation. They invite us to understand the *inclusionary* nature of the new system of care initiated by deinstitutionalisation:

> By inclusionary, we mean a change from the mentally ill being forcibly excluded from society to their being forcibly injected back into society. . . . That is, they are now mostly included in society rather than mostly excluded from it.[20]

Inclusion is not of course synonymous with social integration and as the authors acknowledge the key-notes of what is happening as far as the beneficiaries of policies of inclusion are concerned are ambiguity and uncertainty. Ironically

> mental patients may be more of a mystery today, living among us, than they were when hidden away in the asylum. We do not know them, because they are neither outside society in the world of exclusion, nor are they full citizens – individuals who are like the rest of us. Being neither other or self, they are a new kind of social construction.[21]

This is, indeed, a helpful description of the predicaments of our participants. We may now suggest that one way to characterise the ambiguous kind of social construction that has been brought about by social policies of decarceration and inclusion is as the Person (mental patient) or P(mp) predicament. Formally ex-mental patients in social life are citizens alongside others but in virtue of their history of illness and frequently persisting vulnerability, the entitlement barriers on their participation in social life, and the uncertain reception accorded them, they find themselves placed in an ambiguous and sometimes conflictual relationship with the meanings and consequences that have traditionally attached to the category 'mental patient'. Though bracketed, the category 'mental patient' is none the less still active and the P(mp) predicament may be seen to identify the structurally and culturally unresolved character of the terms of membership and participation available to people with mental illness in social life.

The relevant contrast is with what we may characterise as the Mental Patient (person) predicament or MP(p) in which the person comes to be defined in his or her illness and the category of the person is bracketed but not necessarily abolished – the person may have conferred on him or her the rights and recognitions of what Steven Lukes terms the abstract individual.[22] To state the contrast in this way is to recognise that in so much as it provides space for the re-emergence of the person from under the crippling burden of mental patienthood, the P(mp) predicament is potentially progressive. Yet from the testimonies of our participants, and the wider evidence that is now emerging, it is clear that the accent here is very much on the potential. The message of policy is that people with mental illness are no longer mental patients and have been discharged into the community. But if they are no longer patients then what are they? For some people with mental illness contemporary policy has provided a new set of opportunities but the life chances of others have if anything been degraded still further.

On the available evidence, the transition from the MP(p) to the P(mp) as the representative social predicament for people with mental illness can also plausibly be read as a profoundly retrogressive move in which people with mental illness are returned to the undifferentiated predicaments (joining the ranks of the homeless or the criminal) in which they found themselves in the era before the lunacy reform movement and the construction of the asylums in the nineteenth century. On this reading the P(mp) predicament involves to a considerable extent the reproduction of the marginalisation of people with mental illness under a new set of auspices.

As a number of commentators have shown, for some such people there appears to be no available alternative between mental patienthood and destitution. Homelessness is perhaps the key example of the failure to provide the structures whereby people with mental illness can participate in a manner of ordinary living and it is, indeed, a difficult question to answer as to whether it is preferable to be an unprotected and unhoused ex-mental patient in the community to being a protected mental patient in an asylum. Far from providing access to the entitlements of citizenship for people with mental illness, the Person (mental patient) predicament may equally come to mean that person's health needs are bracketed and all but ignored. This, indeed, is what is suggested by recent evidence about the inability of hard-pressed acute psychiatric services in inner-city areas adequately to address the needs of the homeless mentally ill. If in the recent past complaints were made about the medicalisation of madness, and the incorporation of mentally ill people in total institutions, today under some circumstances people with mental illness find themselves excluded from medical support altogether. It is, perhaps, a bitterly ironic consequence of policies of inclusion that they should have come to generate a social predicament in which people with mental illness may find themselves doubly excluded. If they continue to suffer the negative identification and social exclusion associated with the career mental patient, sometimes in addition they are also excluded from positive identification as people with special needs which require to be addressed.[23]

The product of conflicting impulses (the fiscal crisis of the Welfare State as much as the critiques of institutionalisation), there is therefore not much to celebrate about the P(mp) predicament as we find it.[24] It partakes of conflicts as much as hopes, contains possibilities for good and ill, and as we have seen throws up cruel dilemmas. It is clearly not a unitary phenomenon as much as a family of predicaments that are being worked out within the interacting pressures of the field of forces we have described. In one aspect it seems to promise a solution to old problems, in another it introduces a new set of problems. If people with mental illness have been promised release from the paternalism of psychiatric incorporation, they have at the same time received few of the entitlements and supports necessary to improve their life chances. At stake here is the conflict at the heart of the move from the asylum to the community, remedy for which would presuppose a solution to the wider antagonisms which Dahrendorf has identified. While ex-mental patients and other disadvantaged groups are in possession of certain civil rights, 'until traditional entitlement structures are broken and elements of a civil society created' we cannot legitimately say that they have arrived as citizens, 'they have merely gained a new vantage point in the struggle for more life chances'.[25] 'I hope that the illness will go away', Philip remarked, 'but *they* hope that the person having the illness will go away'. As Dahrendorf enlarges

145

The crucial fact about the underclass and the persistently unemployed is that they have no stake in society. In a very serious sense, society does not need them. Many in the majority class wish that they would simply go away; and if they did their absence would barely be noticed.[26]

Yet it does not follow that we should revert to yesterday's models and seek to reinstate the *ancien régime* of mental patienthood. We do best to view the P(mp) predicament as a marker of where we need to start from, as giving us an indication of where as a society we have now got to in sorting out where people with mental illness belong in social life. Viewed as a conception of how we ought to think rather than as a description of what we actually find, the concept of the Person (mental patient) predicament, in contrast to the frameworks in which people with mental illness have generally been picked up and discussed, does at least convey the ethical commitment to personhood for which we have argued and in these terms can perhaps help to deliver the appropriate conceptions and perspectives from which mental health policy might usefully proceed. If in one light it identifies the tensions and ironies that circumscribe the social fate of the contemporary ex-mental patient, looked at in another we can see that it is in tune with how our participants themselves perceived their situations and wished them to be discussed and addressed.

PSYCHIATRIC SERVICES IN THE COMMUNITY

It may be helpful also to look briefly at the rationalities of psychiatric services in the community within the framework we have sketched and in doing so to locate more firmly the misgivings of many of our participants in their dealings with services.

The conventional wisdom is to conceive the problem in terms of the transfer of patients from a hospital setting to a setting in the community. From this point of view one of the aims of services is to provide for protected forms of participations in social life such as sheltered housing schemes, workschemes, day centres and so forth. Such services may well improve upon the quality of life available to patients under institutional conditions. Equally they may help to mitigate the social forces that would impinge upon patients were they to have to shift for themselves without support. The problem here, however, is that all those awkward questions we have dicussed about the status and worth of ex-mental patients in social life are left unaddressed and not infrequently people are offered a form of protected containment within services which may ease, but do rather little to challenge, the hardships of their structural isolation and serve, as we have seen, only to confirm them in their marginalisation.[27]

Though ex-mental patients in the community may have more opportunities to exercise choice than they did in the asylums, they continue to operate in a context of limited options and resources. In their description of the fate of ex-mental patients in social life in the USA, Dan Lewis and his colleagues presage a development which we may come to see in the United Kingdom in the 'contract culture' of the reformed National Health Service. The ex-mental patient is now commonly described as a consumer but 'it may be more accurate to suggest that such patients have been included in the new mental health system as both commodities and consumers'. Ex-mental patients

have become valuable to service providers in both the public and private sectors by virtue of the money that can be obtained from third parties for their care. After all, the essence of a commodity in the marketplace is that it can be used to generate money as it is processed, improved or simply stored. Patients are used by service providers for this purpose. The movements of patients, therefore, have become the stuff of which markets are made.[28]

In the writers' account of the fortunes of ex-mental patients in the market-place we can identify another twist to the P(mp) predicament:

Patients have some flexibility and power, but it is an odd, negative kind of power – if patients disappear, the ability of the service provider to earn income is in jeopardy. So the patient must stay 'in play', without being a player, caught between the world of income and self-sufficiency and the world of institutions and labels.[29]

One way in which to put the question for psychiatric services is to ask: are they to meet the challenge of the P(mp) predicament on its own terms or are they to reinstate traditional psychiatric paternalisms by conferring on their clients the identity of a community mental patient?

As two commentators have written recently, the 'vision of alternative provision is poorly defined' and there is 'considerable danger that rather than developing new services, the relocation of resources will merely reproduce old services in new places'.[30] Yet if the views of our participants are at all representative, the reproduction of client docility under new auspices is not what is sought after. Michael Ignatieff has nicely characterised the welfare mould from which our participants want in the main to break. The 'citizenship ideal of post-war liberals and social democrats', he writes,

> stressed the passive quality of entitlements at the expense of the active equality of participation. The entitled were never empowered, because empowerment would have infringed the prerogatives of the managers of the welfare state.[31]

As a political question, Ignatieff argues, welfare is about rights not caring. To 'describe the welfare state in the language of caring is to misdescribe it, and to misdescribe is to deceive'. To do so is to reinstate Poor Law principles and to understand the Welfare State as a civic pact between haves and have nots, care-givers and care-receivers, in which entitlements are a matter of moral generosity rather than of right. As Ignatieff aptly remarks, 'only someone who has not actually been on the receiving end of the welfare state would dare call it an instance of civic altruism at work'. Notions of the 'caring society' evoke for Ignatieff 'the image of a nanny state in which the care we get depends on what the "caring professions" think it fit for us to receive'. He would, he goes on, much 'prefer to live in a society which struggles to be just, which respects and enhances people's rights and entitlements'.[32] Simon, we will recall, spoke for many of our participants, when he described how demoralising it felt to be part of the community mental patient system, 'you're sort of tied to the strings of the hospital, the apron strings of the hospital, you're being treated like a child'. As Ignatieff helps us see, the critical issue is not to 'tie us all in the leading strings of therapeutic good intentions' but 'the struggle to make freedom real' through the shared foundation of a 'citizenship of entitlement'.[33]

CULTURAL STYLES OF LIVING WITH MENTAL ILLNESS

To understand some of the problems generated by the community mental patient system we can usefully turn to another American study, *Making It Crazy* by Sue Estroff, based upon two years of fieldwork among people with a history of chronic mental illness in Madison, Wisconsin, and perhaps the most detailed ethnographic study of the lives of people with chronic mental illness in the community yet undertaken.[34] Estroff's book is of interest not only in its own right but also for the differences it throws up from our own inquiry in cultural styles of 'being mentally ill' or living with mental illness. The focus of the study was on forty-three clients in treatment with a community-based programme called PACT (Programme of Assertive Community Treatment), the majority of whom had a diagnosis of schizophrenia. From her exploration of how clients viewed their lives Estroff was led to devise a contrasting typology of 'crazies' and 'normals'. Estroff's use of these categories is ironic and intended to suggest that they are not so much reflections of natural differences between two groups of people as of social and cultural constructions.

In major part her concern is to delineate the creation and perpetuation of a 'mental patient' identity among her client group and to identify the processes that assist in the amplification and maintenance of 'differentness'. What particularly interests Estroff is the way in which people come to accept the 'crazy' identity and to live the 'crazy' life. On Estroff's view 'making it crazy' is a learnt identity which clients come to adopt for lack of any alternative. So, for example, even at the subsistence level – in securing housing, food and other basic requirements – clients find themselves 'enmeshed in a complicated system oriented to psychiatric disability – a system in which their identities or roles as crazy people are the means by which they "make it" or survive'.[35]

The burden of Estroff's argument is that there is no socially available alternative to mental patienthood. The sorts of roles, expectations, stereotypes and responses that are fashioned around long-term psychiatric patients in the community are not markedly different from those that accompany the back-ward patient in the mental hospital. From this point of view, 'simply keeping clients out of the hospital is not enough to stop them and others from "making it crazy"'.[36] As a consequence 'part-time psychotics' living in the community are transformed into 'full-time crazy people'. And if 'crazies' themselves appeared to embrace mental patienthood, 'normals' – including mental health professionals – actively contributed to 'the end result of stabilization within the realm of negative differentness':

> With few exceptions, whichever way we may turn and however we may act in attempts to be helpful, it seems that our psychiatric belief and treatment systems, and our interactions as community members, can contribute not only to the amelioration of patienthood but to its perpetuation. . . . Not only do we describe these persons as pathologically dependent but we contribute to their dependencies. Not only do we view them as unintegrated within the community but we isolate them by constantly

reminding them of their incompetencies and by introducing them to peers (in treatment programs like PACT) with whom they may be more comfortable.[37]

Where in crucial respects Estroff's clients resembled the incorporated, domesticated mental patients of traditional asylum regimes, fashioned in psychiatry's own image, most of our participants were a good deal more combative. In contrast to Estroff's polarities, our inquiry identified a much more differentiated picture that included a number of gradations. So, for example, with perhaps one exception our participants eschewed self-definition as 'crazies' or 'nutters' and to varying degrees, and in different ways, sought to establish and maintain a distance from an identity as a 'mental patient'.

How are we to explain this contrast in identity styles? One explanation is that where Estroff's clients were heavily incorporated in a service system, the services in Northtown were, perhaps, less embracing and offered more opportunities for a distancing from the role of incorporated mental patient. However, it may be that an historical explanation that takes account of the social and cultural matrix in which distinctive cultural styles of living with mental illness, of 'being mentally ill', are formed and negotiated, is also relevant here. Estroff's study was undertaken in the late 1970s and it would appear that in the meantime an increasing number of people with mental illness in western societies have become less enamoured of the roles of domesticated mental patients that had heretofore been offered them. Such changes in cultural style are hinted at in Estroff's most recent work and made explicit in Segal and Baumohl's characterisation of the new generation of chronic mental patients in the USA. These new chronic patients, Segal writes,

> have not been socialised to docility, to the role of acquiescent mental patient; they do not use services in the tractable fashion of their predecessors but rather as wary, often angry, consumers demanding response to their broad needs for social and economic support.[38]

THE CHALLENGE FOR MENTAL HEALTH POLICY

The thrust of our argument in this book has been that in trying to understand the social fate of people with severe mental illness in our society we need to shift the frame of reference from mental patienthood to personhood. To take personhood as the organising principle of our understanding, however, is not to suggest that the problem of mental illness can be abolished. It would be a misrepresentation of the experiences and concerns of our participants to suggest that they could be adequately encompassed in the need for economic and social support. Though our participants did not want to be established in their differences, those differences were, as they themselves recognised, in many cases real enough. Similarly, viewed from the perspective of difference it is evident that people with severe mental illness do not comprise a unitary group. The strategic concerns of Melvin in negotiating the supermarket under the clamour of his voices are clearly somewhat different from those of, say, Ben and Sarah.

Yet as we have tried to show what brings these diverse people together is a shared concern with the terms of membership that are offered them. To deal with them only in their differences without addressing the membership-barriers which exclude them is to do them no service at all. Our characterisation of the Person (mental patient) predicament was an attempt to designate the situation of the person bound by the meanings that attach to a severe mental illness like schizophrenia in our culture and the consequences that flow from them. To transcend the P(mp) predicament as we find it would therefore be to envisage a society in which vulnerability to mental illness did not put the whole of a person's life in question.

Yet on the evidence of our participants it would appear that we have some way to go to achieve this. As we have seen, in their efforts to negotiate their way into a manner of ordinary living contemporary ex-mental patients have, among other things, to battle against versions of psychiatric ideology ('Once a schizophrenic, always a schizophrenic'), professional ideology ('How are you filling your time?') and social prejudice ('Can't trust them with the children'). To remind ourselves of what has gone before, we may conclude with the experience of Ian.

Ian, we recall, had reached a stage where the management of his illness was under control and he was now anxious to identify some form of socially valued project to which he could usefully contribute. On broaching the subject with his consultant, he was disheartened to find that Dr Perkins tried to impress on him a view of himself as only a community mental patient who must be 'content to be on the sick and cope and manage as best' he could. When we asked Ian how he now saw himself, he said: 'Well, I hate myself really'. He then went on to say:

Well, I don't know about hating myself, it's just people's attitudes to mental illness. They won't give you a job, they won't give you any sort of responsibility. I applied to do voluntary work at a place where they look after kids and you go and help out generally, and I applied and told them I had been a student teacher and told them I had had nervous trouble and been in hospital, and they never wrote back and never offered me a position. That was voluntary work!

Ian has made a number of serious suicide attempts in the past and says that he can envisage doing so again. In our judgement, unless some relief can be found for his demoralisation in his struggle for personhood, this is quite a likely outcome.

NOTES

INTRODUCTION

1 On the 'moral careers' of mental patients see, classically, Goffman 1961. For a historical collection of mad people's writings, see Peterson 1982. For an historical study of the voices of the mad see in particular Porter 1987a (see also Porter 1985b and 1988). Studies of the views of 'patients' are beset by theoretical difficulties. For a recent foray here by a psychiatrist see Holloway 1988. For the argument that 'patients' are but the constructs of medicine and their perspectives thereby contaminated see Armstrong 1983, and for a critical discussion within an historical perspective the introduction to Porter 1985a. The most detailed ethnography of ex-mental patients in the community (discussed in Chapter 7) is Estroff 1981; see also Brandon 1981, Davis 1988 and Mangen 1988. An instructive account by a contemporary user of mental health services is Campbell 1989. For a more intemperate collection of such views see Burstow and Weitz 1988. A video-educational package which attempts to give voice to the experiences of people with a history of schizophrenic illness is Barham and Griffiths 1988.

2 Porter 1987a: 35.

3 Porter 1987b: 278.

4 Estroff 1989: 189. Estroff's comments are set within a critical account of this perspective. Estroff argues for an approach which brings the person back into play by means of a conceptual distinction between the 'person' and the 'disorder'. For studies of person–disorder interactions see also Lally 1989 and Strauss 1989. For a complementary conceptualisation of schizophrenia see also Zubin and Spring 1977 and Zubin et al. 1983. For discussion of these issues within an historical perspective on schizophrenia see Barham 1984.

5 Estroff 1989: 191.

6 A helpful critical discussion of 'consumerism' in the mental health sphere is Smith 1989. For a recent attempt to assimilate the perspectives of consumers of mental health services within a professional framework see WHO 1989, and for an empirical study Ritchie et al. 1988. For a discussion of consumer participation largely by consumers themselves see

153

Barker and Peck 1987. A recommendation to practical action based on self-advocacy is Survivors Speak Out 1988.

7 For discussion see Barham 1984, Barham and Hayward 1990, and for the key texts see e.g. Bléuler 1978, Ciompi 1980a and 1980b, Warner 1985 and WHO 1979.

8 See, for discussion, Eisenberg 1988.

9 Porter 1987a: 25.

10 Williams 1962: 117.

11 The participants were located through various formal and informal sources and in assembling the group the following criteria were applied: (1) a definite diagnosis of schizophrenia by Feighner's criteria (Feighner *et al.* 1972); (2) absence of a chronic physical condition; (3) presently residing neither in specialised, staffed accommodation nor with relatives; and (4) knowledge of the diagnosis. The proportion of people with a history of schizophrenic illness living on their own has generally been underestimated. For some recent data on this point see Jones 1988.

12 See, for example, Lewis *et al.* 1989 and Shadish *et al.* 1989.

13 For discussion see Fernando 1988 and Renshaw 1988. For a controversial empirical study see Harrison *et al.* 1988, and for critical comments Fernando 1989. In addition to race, gender merits special attention and illuminating accounts of the experiences of women with mental illness are given in Bachrach and Nadelson 1988.

1 THE PERSON IN QUESTION

1 In the context of the psychiatric culture in which our participants happened to find themselves, Ben's is largely a dissident view. But it is worth remarking that, unbeknown to himself, he makes a cogent case for the vulnerability model of schizophrenia advanced by Zubin and Spring 1977 and Zubin *et al.* 1983.

2 Instructive accounts of the dynamics of reorientation are given in Estroff 1989 and Lally 1989. For discussion of the ways in which people may learn to cope with auditory hallucinations see Romme and Escher 1989. For a helpful discussion of 'living with schizophrenia' within a more conventional social psychiatric framework see Wing 1978. See also Carr 1988.

7 THE PERSON (MENTAL PATIENT) PREDICAMENT

1 For a wide-ranging discussion of how the lives of people with schizophrenia are shaped by political, economic and labour market forces see Warner 1985. For an exploration of the depletion of social networks among ex-mental patients see Gibbons 1983, and for the constraints on 'community' in community care see Bulmer 1987. The testimonies of our participants provide vivid and painful exemplification of the accounts of stigma and 'spoiled identity' in Goffman 1963 and Freidson 1970. As Freidson summarises it: 'identity is formed by the fact of *having* been in a stigmatized role: the cured mental patient is not just another person but an ex-mental patient. . . . One's identity is permanently spoiled' (1970: 236).

2   Strauss 1989: 182.
3   Strauss 1989: 184.
4   Estroff 1989: 191.
5   Estroff 1989: 191.
6   Estroff 1989: 194.
7   Taylor 1989: 23.
8   Taylor 1989: 34.
9   Taylor 1989: 112.
10 Taylor 1989: 28.
11 Taylor 1989: 42, 44.
12 Taylor 1989: 42.
13 Taylor 1989: 44.
14 Taylor 1989: 47.
15 Taylor 1989: 47.
16 Taylor 1989: 52.
17 Harris 1985: 25.
18 Dahrendorf 1988: 152. On poverty in the British context see, for example, Townsend 1986.
19 Dahrendorf 1988: 37.
20 Lewis *et al.* 1989: 173–4. For an account of the conflicting meanings of deinstitutionalisation see Bachrach 1989.
21 Lewis *et al.* 1989: 173–4.
22 Lukes 1973: 152–3.
23 On the homeless mentally ill in the USA see Torrey 1989, and on discharged mental patients in London Kay and Legg 1986. An account of pressure on acute psychiatric services in an inner-city area is Patrick *et al.* 1989.
24 For discussion of the fiscal crisis of the Welfare State as it affects mental health policies see Scull 1984. On health and deprivation see Townsend *et al.* 1988a and 1988b, and for discussion of the social fate of people with chronic illness generally Anderson and Bury 1988.
25 Dahrendorf 1988: 14, 47.
26 Dahrendorf 1988: 161.
27 Farkas and Anthony 1989 provide a telling summary of the position in the USA: 'Research, simply put, tells us that the mental health system has been unable to convince many psychiatrically disabled clients to accept and remain in community based treatment. 50–66% of those referred for aftercare services did not show up. Of those who did, 40% stopped coming after one session' (1989: 178). A helpful account of day services in Britain is Carter 1981. It would, of course, be quite misleading to suggest that alternative forms of service have not been proposed and in some cases developed. See e.g. Brackx and Grimshaw 1989, Braisby *et al.* 1988, Lavender and Holloway 1988, MIND 1989, Patmore 1987 and Ramon 1988.
28 Lewis *et al.* 1989: 178.
29 Lewis *et al.* 1989: 178.
30 Towell and Kingsley 1988: 171.
31 Ignatieff 1989: 69.
32 Ignatieff 1989: 70–1.

33 Ignatieff 1989: 72, 74.
34 Estroff 1981, but see especially 1985 edition with update.
35 Estroff 1981: 38.
36 Estroff 1981: 254.
37 Estroff 1981: 174.
38 Segal and Baumohl 1985: 112.

REFERENCES

Anderson, R. and Bury, M. (eds) (1988) *Living with Chronic Illness*, London: Unwin Hyman.

Armstrong, D. (1983) *The Political Anatomy of the Body*, Cambridge: Cambridge University Press.

Bachrach, L. (1989) 'Deinstitutionalization: a semantic analysis', *Journal of Social Issues* 45 (3), 161–71.

Bachrach, L. and Nadelson, C. C. (eds) (1988) *Treating Chronically Mentally Ill Women*, Washington, DC: American Psychiatric Press.

Barham, P. (1984) *Schizophrenia and Human Value*, Oxford: Basil Blackwell.

Barham, P. and Griffiths, G. (eds) (1988) *Beyond the Hospital: A Video Educational Package*, Brighton: Pavilion Publishing.

Barham, P. and Hayward, R. (1990) 'Schizophrenia as a life-process', in R. Bentall (ed.) *Reconstructing Schizophrenia*, London: Routledge.

Barker, I. and Peck, E. (eds) (1987) *Power in Strange Places*, London: Good Practices in Mental Health.

Bleuler, M. (1978) *The Schizophrenic Disorders*, New Haven, Conn.: Yale University Press (first published 1972 as *Die Schizophrenen Geistesstorungen im Lichte Langjahrige Kranken und Familiengeschichten*, Stuttgart: Georg Thieme).

Brackx, A. and Grimshaw, C. (eds) (1989) *Mental Health Care in Crisis*, London: Pluto Press.

Braisby, D., Echlin, R., Hill, S. and Smith, S. (1988) *Changing Futures: Housing and Support Services for People Discharged from Psychiatric Hospitals*, London: King's Fund.

Brandon, D. (1981) *Voices of Experience: Consumer Perspectives on Psychiatric Treatment*, London: MIND Publications.

Bulmer, M. (1987) *The Social Basis of Community Care*, London: Unwin.

Burstow, B. and Weitz, D. (eds) (1988) *Shrink Resistant*, Vancouver: New Star.

Campbell, P. (1989) 'Peter Campbell's story', in A. Brackx and C. Grimshaw (eds) *Mental Health Care in Crisis*, London: Pluto Press.

Carr, V. (1988) 'Patients' techniques for coping with schizophrenia: an exploratory study', *British Journal of Medical Psychology* 61 (4), 339–52.

Carter, J. (1981) *Day Services for Adults*, London: Allen & Unwin.

Ciompi, L. (1980a) 'Ist die chronische Schizophrenie ein Artefakt? Argumente

157

und Gegenargumente', *Fortschritte der Neurologie-Psychiatrie* (Stuttgart) 48, 237–48.

——(1980b) 'The natural history of schizophrenia in the long term', *British Journal of Psychiatry* 136, 413–20.

Dahrendorf, R. (1988) *The Modern Social Conflict*, London: Weidenfeld & Nicolson.

Davis, A. (1988) 'User's perspectives', in S. Ramon (ed.) *Psychiatry in Transition*, London: Pluto Press.

Eisenberg, L. (1988) 'The social construction of mental illness', *Psychological Medicine* 18, 1–9.

Estroff, S. (1981) *Making it Crazy*, Berkeley, Calif.: University of California Press (revised paperback edn 1985).

—— (1989) 'Self, identity, and the subjective experiences of schizophrenia', *Schizophrenia Bulletin* 15 (2), 189–96.

Farkas, M. and Anthony, W. (1989) 'Psychiatric rehabilitation: fiction or fact?' in H. von Hippius, H. Lauter, D. Ploog, H. Bieber and L. van Hout (eds) *Rehabilitation in der Psychiatrie*, Berlin: Springer-Verlag.

Feighner, J., Robins, E., Guze, S., Woodruff, R., Winokur, G. and Munoz, R. (1972) 'The diagnostic criteria for use in psychiatric research', *Archives of General Psychiatry* 26, 57–63.

Fernando, S. (1988) *Race and Culture in Psychiatry*, London: Croom Helm.

——(1989) 'Letter', *Psychiatric Bulletin* 13 (10) 573–4.

Freidson, E. (1970) *Profession of Medicine*, New York: Dodd, Mead.

Gibbons, J. (1983) *Care of Schizophrenic Patients in the Community*, third annual report, Department of Psychiatry, University of Southampton.

Goffman, E. (1961) *Asylums*, Harmondsworth: Penguin.

——(1963) *Stigma*, Harmondsworth: Penguin.

Harris, J. (1985) *The Value of Life*, London: Routledge & Kegan Paul.

Harrison, G., Owens, D., Holton, A., Neilson, D. and Boot, D. (1988) 'A prospective study of severe mental disorder in Afro-Caribbean patients', *Psychological Medicine* 18, 643–57.

Holloway, F. (1988) 'Psychiatric day-care: the users' perspective', *International Journal of Social Psychiatry* 35 (3) 252–64.

Ignatieff, M. (1989) 'Citizenship and moral narcissism', *Political Quarterly* 60 (1), 63–74.

Jones, K. (1988) 'Schizophrenia tracer project: report on stage one', unpublished, Department of Social Policy and Social Work, University of York.

Kay, A. and Legg, C. (1986) *Discharged to the Community*, London: Good Practices in Mental Health.

Lally, S. (1989) 'Does being in here mean there's something wrong with me?', *Schizophrenia Bulletin* 15 (2), 253–66.

Lavender, A. and Holloway, F. (eds) (1988) *Community Care in Practice*, London: Wiley.

Lewis, D., Shadish, W. and Lurigio, A. (1989) 'Policies of inclusion and the mentally ill: long-term care in a new environment', *Journal of Social Issues* 45 (3), 173–86.

Lukes, S. (1973) *Individualism*, Oxford: Basil Blackwell.

Mangen, S. (1988) 'Dependence or autonomy', in S. Ramon (ed.) *Psychiatry in Transition*, London: Pluto Press.

MIND (1989) *Building Better Futures*, London: MIND Publications.

Patmore, C. (ed.) (1987) *Living after Mental Illness*, London: Croom Helm.

Patrick, M., Higgit, A. and Holloway, F. (1989) 'Changes in an inner-city psychiatric in-patient service', *Health Trends* 21, 121–3.

Peterson, D. (ed.) (1982) *A Mad People's History of Madness*, Pittsburgh: University of Pittsburgh Press.

Porter, R. (ed.) (1985a) *Patients and Practitioners*, Cambridge: Cambridge University Press.

——(1985b) 'The hunger of imagination: approaching Samuel Johnson's melancholy', in W. Bynum, R. Porter and M. Shepherd (eds) *The Anatomy of Madness*, vol. I, London: Tavistock.

——(1987a) *The Social History of Madness*, London: Weidenfeld & Nicolson.

——(1987b) 'Bedlam and Parnassus: mad people's writing in Georgian England', in G. Levine (ed.) *One Culture*, Wisonsin: University of Wisconsin Press.

——(1988) 'Margery Kempe and the meaning of madness', *History Today* 38, 39–44.

Ramon, S. with Giannichedda, M. (1988) *Psychiatry in Transition*, London: Pluto Press.

Renshaw, J. (1988) *Mental Health Care to Ethnic Minority Groups*, London: Good Practices in Mental Health.

Ritchie, J., Morrissey, C. and Ward, K. (1988) '*Keeping in Touch with the Talking*', Research Report I, Birmingham Community Care Special Action Project.

Romme, M. and Escher, A. (1989) 'Hearing Voices', *Schizophrenia Bulletin* 15 (2), 209–16.

Scull, A. (1984) *Decarceration*, 2nd edn, Oxford: Polity Press (first published 1977 Englewood Cliffs, NJ: Prentice-Hall).

Segal, S. and Baumohl, J. (1985) 'The community living-room', *Journal of Contemporary Social Work* Feb., 111–16.

Shadish, W., Lugurio, A. and Lewis, D. (1989) 'After deinstitutionalization: the present and future of mental health long-term care policy', *Journal of Social Issues* 45 (3), 1–15.

Smith, H. (1989) 'Collaboration for change: partnership between service users, planners and managers of mental health services', in D. Towell, S. Kingsley and T. McAusland (eds) *Managing Psychiatric Services in Transition*, London: King's Fund.

Strauss, J. (1989) 'Subjective experiences of schizophrenia: towards a new dynamic psychiatry II', *Schizophrenia Bulletin* 15 (2), 179–88.

Survivors Speak Out (1989) *Self-Advocacy Action Pack*, Survivors Speak Out, 41 Kenwyn Drive, London NW2 7NX.

Taylor, C. (1989) *Sources of the Self*, Cambridge: Cambridge University Press.

Torrey, E. F. (1989) *Nowhere to go: The Tragic Odyssey of the Homeless Mentally Ill*, New York: Harper & Row.

Towell, D. and Kingsley, S. (1988) 'Changing psychiatric services in Britain', in S. Ramon with M. Giannichedda (eds) *Psychiatry in Transition*, London: Pluto Press.

Townsend, P. (1986) 'Why are the many poor?', *International Journal of Health Services* 16 (1): 1–32.

Townsend, P., Davidson, N. and Whitehead, M. (eds) (1988a) *Inequalities in Health*, Harmondsworth: Penguin.

Townsend, P., Phillimore, P. and Beattie, A. (1988b) *Health and Deprivation*, London: Croom Helm.

Warner, R. (1985) *Recovery from Schizophrenia*, London: Routledge & Kegan Paul.

WHO (1979) *Schizophrenia: An International Follow-up Study*, London: Wiley.

——(1989) *Consumer Involvement in Mental Health and Rehabilitation Services* (WHO/MNH/MEP, 89.7) Geneva: Division of Mental Health, World Health Organization.

Williams, B. (1962) 'The idea of equality', in P. Laslett and W. G. Runciman (eds) *Philosophy, Politics and Society* (2nd Series), Oxford: Basil Blackwell.

Wing, J. K. (1978) 'Social influence on the course of schizophrenia', in L. Wynne, R. Cromwell and S. Matthysse (eds) *The Nature of Schizophrenia*, New York: Wiley.

Zubin, J., Magaziner, J. and Steinhauer, S. (1983) 'The metamorphosis of schizophrenia: from chronicity to vulnerability', *Psychological Medicine* 13, 551–71.

Zubin, J. and Spring, B. (1977) 'Vulnerability: a new view of schizophrenia', *Journal of Abnormal Psychology* 86, 103–26.

INDEX

161